Short essay questions for MRCOG Part 2

For Churchill Livingstone:

Commissioning editors: Timothy Horne
Project editor: Barbara Simmons
Production controller: Nancy Arnott
Design direction: Sarah Cape

Short Essay Questions for MRCOG Part 2

M.A. Khaled MBBS LMSSA MRCOG
Senior Registrar, Obstetrics and Gynaecology, Wythenshawe Hospital,
Manchester, UK

A.G. Ellis MB ChB MRCOG
Senior Registrar, Obstetrics and Gynaecology, Hope Hospital, Manchester, UK

With a chapter on the oral assessment examination by

Pamela Buck FRCOG
Senior Lecturer, Department of Obstetrics and Gynaecology,
University of Manchester, UK
Member Part 2 MRCOG Oral Assessment Subcommittee RCOG
Formerly Chairman, OSCE Subcommittee RCOG

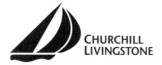
CHURCHILL
LIVINGSTONE

EDINBURGH LONDON NEW YORK PHILADELPHIA SYDNEY TORONTO 1999

CHURCHILL LIVINGSTONE
An imprint of Harcourt Brace and Company Limited

Churchill Livingstone, 1-3 Baxter's Place, Leith Walk, Edinburgh EH1 3AF

© Harcourt Brace and Company Limited 1999

🦢 is a registered trademark of Harcourt Brace and Company Limited.

ISBN 0443 061963

British Library of Cataloguing in Publication Data
A catalogue record for this book is available from the British Library.

Library of Congress Cataloging in Publication Data
A catalog record for this book is available from the Library of Congress.

Medical knowledge is constantly changing. As information becomes available,
changes in treatment, procedures, equipment and the use of drugs become
necessary. The author and publisher have, as far as it is possible, taken care to
ensure that the information given in the text is accurate and up-to-date. However,
readers are strongly advised to confirm that the information, especially with regard to
drug usage, complies with current legislation and standard of practice.

The
publisher's
policy is to use
paper manufactured
from sustainable forests

Printed by Bell and Bain Ltd., Glasgow

Preface

This book is aimed at those candidates preparing for the Part 2 MRCOG examination. As the authors are actively involved in Part 2 teaching, the book was conceived in response to the evident uncertainty (and in some candidates despair) produced by the change in the examination format! The short essays require a different technique to the old format long essays. Time management and the writing of a well-structured, concise answer is crucial. Unfortunately, this only comes with practice. Most candidates who fail the written section berate themselves for not knuckling down to actual timed essay practice. Finding a senior to provide good feedback is not always easy and motivation is hard when you have been up all night CTG watching. The aim of this book is to try to make essay practice a little less painful.

The oral assessment examination has been embraced by medical schools and has been central to the DRCOG for some time now. Those with a sound clinical background should romp through the MRCOG oral assessment examination, provided they play the game according to the rules. Pam Buck outlines a common sense approach to the examination.

We have not forgotten the agonies of the MRCOG and our aim is that you should only have to endure it once!

1999   M.K.
                                                                                A.E.

Acknowledgements

We would particularly like to acknowledge the help and guidance given to us by Roger Jackson, the RCOG examination secretary, which kept us on track. We would also like to express our appreciation of the secretarial effort of Chris Laing, who painstakingly checked and corrected the manuscript.

Of course this book would not have been possible without the tolerance of our respective spouses (Sarra and Simon) and our children (Heba, Ahmed, Christopher and Alexander).

Contents

Answering the short essay paper

EXAMINATION PREPARATION

Remember there is no point in panicking. If you have done the correct preparation, you will pass! If you have not, either don't do the examination or go with a positive attitude.

6 months beforehand

Book a place on a suitable revision course. Arrange duties so that you have no on-call commitments for at least 3 days before the examination. If you are able, take holiday or study leave for 1 week before the examination date. Read a copy of the examination regulations.

The major mistake candidates make with their examination preparation is not to keep their finger on the pulse of current affairs. Don't base all your revision round traditional textbooks.

Aim to cover the recent (last 2 years of) mainstream British journals e.g.:

- *British Journal of Obstetrics and Gynaecology*
- *Journal of Obstetrics and Gynaecology*
- *Lancet* and *BMJ*
- *British Journal of Hospital Medicine*
- *Current Obstetrics and Gynaecology.*

Remember that some are available not only in the library but also on the Internet, for those of you who are computer literate!

Although the above should form the core of your reading, do read other journals of interest. Most important of these are the American journals. Care must be taken with overseas journals. Make sure that they do not confuse your perception of practice in the UK.

For current affairs, read the broadsheet newspapers, medical press such as *Hospital Doctor*, and the editorials and news pages of the above journals. When revising from textbooks, it is more productive to use active learning rather than aiming to read a textbook cover to cover. Use a book of multiple choice questions (MCQs) to assess your level of knowledge and target your textbook reading to remedy areas of weakness. If you see an interesting case in clinical practice, go and read the appropriate textbook reference. This will reinforce your learning and ensure long-term retention of facts.

Make very *brief* revision notes on the areas you find difficult (for example, the up-to-date FIGO staging for gynaecological malignancies).

Don't forget your preparation for the new RCOG oral assessment examination. Make sure that, between the written examination and the oral assessment examination, you continue revising. Although difficult, do not wait for the results, as otherwise revision time is wasted.

Practise short essays! Practice makes perfect!

1 month beforehand

Book accommodation and complete travel plans. Make these as foolproof as possible. Take into account traffic and parking. If necessary, stay in a hotel within walking distance of the examination.

Work on MCQs, short essay practice and targeted learning.

Keep up to date with your chosen journals.

Learn and relearn your 'difficult' topics from your prepared revision notes.

Day before the examination

1. Check your equipment! RCOG identification card (or other identification document which includes name and photograph), directions and details. Check pens etc. Make sure you have a spare!
2. If in an unfamiliar place, visit the site of the examination so that there is no chance of getting lost on the day. Make sure that you have an accurate idea of the travel time in traffic and make parking arrangements.

Go to bed early!

THE EXAMINATION

The instructions to candidates for the Part 2 MRCOG Examination are as follows:

Instructions to candidates

Read these instructions carefully before answering any questions.
Write your candidate number on each sheet.

- You have **two** hours to complete the five short answers.
- The answers should demonstrate your *critical* understanding of recent ideas in obstetrics and gynaecology.
- **Do not write lists or short notes.**
- You may **only** use one sheet of paper for each question but may use both sides.
- **No** extra paper/additional sheets will be provided.
- Rough notes can be made on the coloured paper provided.
- **Do not remove any sheets from this booklet.**

No matter how many times you have sat the examination, *read the instructions* thoroughly. Then *read the essay titles* through. Start with *the easiest question*. This is not just a good psychological boost. As with most examinations, the key to success is *time management*. By starting with the easiest question, this allows you to settle in quickly and focus on the task ahead. It also allows you to accumulate spare time that can be allocated at the end to the more difficult questions. Remember to keep your mind focused only on the question in hand.

Having decided on where to start, *read the question, then read the question again.*

Analyse the wording

Here are some possibilities of phrasing of essay questions. During your examination preparation, make sure that you understand exactly what is required of each. If you encounter a different phrase, we would suggest adding this to the list below. Terms such as 'discuss' or 'debate' can indicate the need for quite lengthy answers and therefore are rarely used in this format. If used, these terms are likely to be qualified: for example, briefly debate.

Explain	Formulate
Debate	Outline
Discuss	Critically appraise
Evaluate	How would you approach?
Compare and contrast	Consider the options
Critically	Explore
Discuss changes, controversies	Give a detailed account
or advances	How would you proceed?
What advice or how would you advise?	How would you counsel?
Briefly debate	Describe
Summarise	Compare
Justify	How would you investigate?
Review	

Next, look at the content of the question. Decide what needs to be included in your answer. For example, a mental checklist for an obstetric question would be preconceptual (prenatal), antenatal (first, second, third trimester), intrapartum, postpartum.

If the question includes management, unless stated otherwise, history, examination, investigation, treatment and follow-up must be covered.

Answering the question

Write a very short plan on the sheet of rough paper provided. *Do not* use the rough paper to write the answer with the intention of copying it out in best. This is far too time-consuming.

Be very disciplined and concise with the answer. Remember that the ideal answer should be around 250 words (one side) and certainly must be no longer than 450 words (two sides). Make sure that every point is clear: do not assume that your examiner can automatically follow your train of thought and draw the same conclusions.

Remember that the answer must take the form of a *short essay*, not short notes. So essay style is essential.

Take care that handwriting is legible. Sometimes at the end of the essay paper, a bit of extra mental effort is required to do this! Once again, leaving enough time and concentrating on giving a concise answer will help with your handwriting. When crossing out a sentence, put brackets round it and then cross out with a single firm line.

The maximum time allowed per question is 24 minutes. Therefore, guillotine your answers at 20 minutes. Move on to the next question and return at the end of the examination if you have enough time.

   The difficult question at the end.   Don't panic. It is likely that if you don't like the question, then most of the other candidates won't like it either! Hopefully you are secure in the knowledge that you have made a reasonable attempt at the rest of the paper and that you have left adequate time to give a carefully thought out answer. Analyse the wording of the question carefully. Are there any clues that you have missed? Try to categorise your answer, for example anatomically, as in vulval, vaginal, cervical, uterine, fallopian or ovarian causes of postmenopausal bleeding. Still stuck where to start? Think how you have dealt with a similar problem. What would you say to your Senior House Officer or medical student? Imagine what you would say to a patient during counselling.

HOW TO USE THIS BOOK

There are three ways of using this book:

1. *As mock examinations.* Use a systematic approach, performing one paper a week over the preceding 6 months. This is because the points regarding examination technique, made after each answer, tend to build up through the book. For at least the last 2 months, we recommend answering the papers against the clock. After answering the paper, this should be followed by targeted revision of the topics included. In particular, read the suggested reading. This has been kept purposefully short, preferentially includes review articles and where possible the most accessible references have been used.
2. *As a spotter.* This book has been made of a handy size so that it is easily portable. So it can be used to self-test your knowledge/your approach to a question when waiting to do that critical V/E on call.
3. *As an aid to topic revision.* In this approach, question answering is used to test the adequacy of revision of a topic. This is only effective if you then revise the topic again to remedy any deficiencies and reinforce learning. Unless, of course, you have produced the perfect answer!

We consider the first option to be the best, but the choice is yours.

OBSTETRICS

Obstetrics questions

1. Pregnant women receive 'too much' antenatal care. Critically appraise this statement.

2. A woman has previously had an unexplained stillbirth at 41 weeks' gestation. She now presents at 32 weeks' gestation in a planned second pregnancy, wishing to discuss her anxieties regarding the remainder of her obstetric care. Justify your management.

3. A woman presents with a term twin pregnancy in labour. Following the delivery of the first twin, the second is found to be lying transversely. Justify your approach to delivery of the second twin.

4. A 38-year-old primigravid woman suffers from familial hyperlipidaemia and angina. She presents at 30 weeks' gestation with a singleton pregnancy, in early labour. Discuss optimal intrapartum management.

5. Following a prolonged first labour and instrumental delivery, a 30-year-old woman continues to trickle blood per vaginum. Outline your management plan.

PAPER 2

1. Critically evaluate antenatal booking investigations.

2. A 22-year-old unbooked African woman presents at 24 weeks' gestation with abdominal pain. How would you reach a diagnosis?

3. After a normal vertex delivery of a healthy full-term infant, the woman collapses. How would you manage this obstetric problem?

4. A primigravida presents at 32 weeks' gestation with confirmed spontaneous rupture of membranes (SROM). Justify your management.

5. Following an uneventful pregnancy, a primigravid woman presents at 42 weeks' gestation. Compare and contrast the management options available.

PAPER 3

1. Caesarean section can be justified on maternal request alone. Debate this statement.

2. A 32-year-old parous woman presents at the booking clinic with a history of severe postnatal depression after her last delivery. Outline your approach to her care.

3. Following an uneventful twin pregnancy, a routine ultrasound scan examination shows fetal death of one twin in utero. Justify your management.

4. Describe the intrapartum complications that are associated with a diabetic pregnancy at 38 weeks' gestation and discuss possible methods of prevention.

5. A 39-year-old woman conceives following infertility treatment. A routine ultrasound at 16 weeks reveals a quadruplet pregnancy. How would you counsel her?

PAPER 4

1. Critically appraise the input of multidisciplinary clinics into obstetric care.

2. Having recently returned from a holiday abroad, a woman presents at 28 weeks' gestation with a persistent pyrexia of unknown origin and abdominal pain. How would you reach a diagnosis?

3. A woman was involved in a road traffic accident at 26 weeks' gestation. Discuss the obstetric contribution to her care.

4. Following a prolonged labour, a 17-year-old primiparous patient delivers a healthy 4050 g baby vaginally and subsequently has a massive postpartum haemorrhage. Discuss the priorities in the management of this obstetric emergency.

5. A primigravida presents with an unexplained stillbirth at 37 weeks' gestation. Review the psychological aspects of her care.

PAPER 5

1. Evaluate the role of maternal serum screening for Down syndrome.

2. A 30-year-old woman is known to be HIV-positive and is now 14 weeks' pregnant. Review the implications of her serostatus for her obstetric care.

3. A 28-year-old nulliparous woman has long-standing insulin-dependent diabetes mellitus (IDDM) and is known to have renal impairment secondary to diabetic nephropathy. She states her wish to plan a family. How would you counsel her?

4. A primigravida presents at term with a persistent occipitoposterior position and failure to progress in the second stage of labour. How would you select an appropriate method of delivery?

5. During an artificial rupture of membranes (ARM) at 8 cm cervical dilatation, sudden bleeding was associated with a profound fetal bradycardia. Give a detailed account of your management.

PAPER 6

1. A 27-year-old renal transplant recipient is contemplating a pregnancy. How would you counsel her?

2. A 23-year-old who had a forceps delivery is found to have had a third-degree tear. Give a detailed account of your management.

3. A successful amniocentesis of one of two gestation sacs shows that the chromosomal pattern is consistent with Edward's syndrome, while the other fetus has a normal karyotype. Critically discuss the management options.

4. The labour ward statistics reveal that the caesarean section rate at your hospital has climbed over 5 years from 12% to 25%. How would you address this problem?

5. Outline the management of a singleton small-for-dates pregnancy at 30 weeks' gestation for the remainder of the pregnancy.

PAPER 7

1. Compare and contrast the methods used in invasive prenatal diagnosis.

2. Following an uneventful singleton pregnancy, a woman presents at the antenatal clinic at 36 weeks' gestation. She has one other child born by caesarean section, owing to failure to progress in labour. Justify how you would reach a decision regarding her mode of delivery.

3. A primigravida with a multiple pregnancy attends for a routine antenatal visit at 34 weeks' gestation. Her blood pressure is found to be 160/100 mmHg and urinalysis reveals 2 g of protein. Justify your management.

4. A primiparous woman has a stillbirth at 36 weeks' gestation. Evaluate the investigations available.

5. Following two first trimester miscarriages, a 27-year-old woman presents at 8 weeks' gestation at the antenatal booking clinic. On examination, she is noted to have a goitre and exophthalmos. Explore further management.

PAPER 8

1. How valuable is the obstetric day care unit in current obstetric practice?

2. An ultrasound scan examination at 24 weeks' gestation shows ascites and confirms fetal death in utero. How would you investigate the cause of this? Justify your answer.

3. A parous woman presents at 38 weeks' gestation with a confirmed singleton breech presentation. She requests a vaginal breech delivery. How would you assess whether this mode of delivery would be feasible?

4. A 35-year-old woman presents at 30 weeks' gestation in her second pregnancy for a routine antenatal visit. It is noted that 3 years previously she had a subarachnoid haemorrhage. Debate your management.

5. A 30-year-old parous woman is referred by her general practitioner at 27 weeks' gestation with jaundice. Account for your strategy to reach a diagnosis.

PAPER 9

1. An obese 35-year-old primigravida is found to have two episodes of glycosuria in the second trimester. Justify your approach to the management of the remainder of her pregnancy.

2. Critically review the role of ultrasound scan examination in modern obstetrics.

3. An unbooked 26-year-old woman presents in advanced labour at term. She admits to a history of drug addiction. How would you conduct her care?

4. Review the principles and recent developments regarding rhesus prophylaxis.

5. Compare and contrast the anticonvulsant agents available for the prevention of eclamptic fits.

PAPER 10

1. At 30 weeks' gestation, an ultrasound scan examination reveals a major degree of placenta praevia. Justify your management plan for the remainder of the pregnancy.

2. What information do you gain from macroscopic examination of a placenta?

3. At 34 weeks' gestation, a primigravida presents with a generalised seizure. Outline your proposed management.

4. A 35-year-old presents with excessive vomiting and 8 weeks' amenorrhoea. Discuss your management.

5. Following an uneventful antenatal course, a routine full blood count at 28 weeks' gestation reveals a platelet count of $56 \times 10^9/L$. Formulate a management plan for the remainder of the pregnancy.

Obstetrics answers

1. **Pregnant women receive 'too much' antenatal care. Critically appraise this statement.**

The recent push for change in the organisation of the maternity services was originally detailed in the government publication 'Changing Childbirth'. The call for a re-evaluation and possible reduction of the number of routine antenatal visits was one of the recommendations that emerged. The role of improving social and economic factors in reducing perinatal mortality and morbidity is not in dispute. The contribution of modern antenatal care is more difficult to evaluate and there have been no studies that have satisfactorily answered this question.

Those women with 'high risk' pregnancies undoubtedly do not receive too much antenatal care as the level of parental anxiety, in addition to the requirements for monitoring of the pregnancy, dictates the number of antenatal visits. Several visits may be required, not only to gain rapport with the prospective parents, but also to discuss more complicated points and to adequately counsel some couples. However, improved use of multidisciplinary clinics may decrease the total number of hospital visits in these pregnancies.

The major part of the demand on antenatal services results from the care of low-risk pregnancy. The current model of antenatal care in cases of low-risk pregnancy is criticised not only on grounds of cost-effectiveness, but by making normal pregnancy a 'disease' rather than a physiological process. On the other hand, frequent antenatal visits allow a rapport to develop (provided some continuity of care is assured) and allow some parentcraft discussion to be initiated. The psychological support provided by antenatal visits needs to be more fully evaluated.

In conclusion, 'low-risk pregnancies' probably do receive more antenatal visits than can be justified purely on *cost-effective* grounds. However, in the absence of a method of reliably identifying these low-risk women, it is not currently possible to provide a more woman-centred approach. Until targeting of antenatal care is possible, devolving of more 'routine' antenatal care to the primary care team will improve cost-effectiveness, allow combination with parentcraft sessions and should be more acceptable to women in terms of accessibility. Emphasis should be placed on the *quality rather than the quantity* of antenatal visits.

Comments

This is a topical question and mentioning the 'Changing Childbirth' report demonstrates your knowledge of current affairs. This question illustrates the importance of keeping up to date with medical news. Talk to your consultants about hot issues. Business managers and midwifery managers are also a good source of information.

The use of 'politically correct' terms (woman-centred approach, cost-effective, high-risk and low-risk pregnancy, primary care team, accessibility, multidisciplinary clinics) also demonstrates knowledge of current affairs.

This is a question in which waffling is far too easy. Keep the answer tightly to the brief plan that you have written on the piece of rough paper.

Suggested reading

Department of Health 1993 Changing childbirth. Report of the Expert Maternity Group. HMSO, London

Enkin M, Kierse M J N C 1989 Vol 1: Pregnancy. In: Chalmers I (ed) Effective care in pregnancy and childbirth. Oxford University Press, Oxford

Hall M, Chang P K, MacGillivary I 1980 Is routine antenatal care worthwhile? Lancet 2: 78–80

Pearson V 1994 Frequency and timing of antenatal visits. Health Care Evaluation Unit, University of Bristol, Bristol

Renfrew M J 1997 Influencing the development of evidence-based practice. British Journal of Midwifery 5(3): 131–134

Royal College of Obstetricians and Gynaecologists 1995 Report of Joint Working Group on Organisational Standards for Maternity Services. RCOG, London

2. **A woman has previously had an unexplained stillbirth at 41 weeks' gestation. She now presents at 32 weeks' gestation in a planned second pregnancy, wishing to discuss her anxieties regarding the remainder of her obstetric care. Justify your management.**

Careful counselling of the woman and her partner is essential. Adequate time must be allocated to do this and privacy afforded.

The risk of recurrent stillbirth is only slightly increased, but attention must be focused on possible recurrent causes of stillbirth, and the current pregnancy must be managed as 'high risk'. Although the previous stillbirth was 'unexplained', the possibility of placental insufficiency or gestational diabetes must be considered, as this was a post-term loss.

The antenatal progress in the current pregnancy must be reviewed and clinical examination performed. In this high-risk pregnancy, ultrasound scan examination, cardiotocography and Doppler assessment of the umbilical cord is justified. Fetal growth, liquor volume and cardiotocography are the best prognostic indicators and, if normal, a formal biophysical profile is unlikely to provide any additional information. This assessment can be repeated at fortnightly intervals. If glucose intolerance is suspected, a glucose tolerance test is appropriate.

Although relatively late in pregnancy, it is important to advise the woman to avoid risk factors for stillbirth, such as smoking or taking of illicit drugs. The benefit of formal kick charts is unproven, but the woman should be told to monitor fetal movements and contact the unit if concerned.

The timing and mode of delivery will be judged in relation to the perceived risk to the fetus. Preterm delivery of a compromised fetus would be undertaken after consultation with paediatric colleagues. Prior to 34 weeks' gestation, antenatal steroids should be administered to produce fetal lung maturation. If the current pregnancy is healthy, the suspicion of possible placental insufficiency in the first pregnancy is still an indication for delivery prior to the expected date of confinement. This may also be of psychological benefit to the couple. A few women prefer no medical intervention, in which case 'watchful waiting' can be employed. The mode of delivery is based on both obstetric criteria and the wishes of the couple. In cases of intrapartum loss, previous caesarean section or with evidence of fetal compromise, delivery by caesarean section may be considered. Otherwise, induction of labour can be undertaken if spontaneous labour does not intervene.

Comments

In this question, counselling is obviously a central issue and your answer must emphasise this. Management does, however, also include history, examination, investigation and treatment (in this case, delivery).

This is actually a straightforward question, but the key is to be disciplined in your approach. Stick to your time limit of 20 minutes.

Suggested reading

Chamberlain G (ed) 1995 Turnbull's obstetrics. Churchill Livingstone, Edinburgh

Enkin M, Kierse M J N C 1989 Vol 1: Pregnancy. In: Chalmers I (ed) Effective care in pregnancy and childbirth. Oxford University Press, Oxford

James D K, Steer P J, Weiner C P, Gonik B (eds) 1994 High risk pregnancy – management options. Saunders, London

3. **A woman presents with a term twin pregnancy in labour. Following the delivery of the first twin, the second is found to be lying transversely. Justify your approach to delivery of the second twin.**

The obstetric aim is to deliver the second twin within 20 minutes of the first, as the risk of placental separation increases markedly after this time. With this in mind, the anaesthetist, as well as the paediatricians, should be present on the labour ward in case an operative delivery is required.

If the membranes of the second twin are still intact, the lie can be converted to longitudinal. Initially, external cephalic version would be attempted, followed by a controlled rupture of the membranes with the onset of the next uterine contraction. If required, the delivery can be expedited using the vacuum extractor. Should the external approach be unsuccessful, there are two options: either to perform internal podalic version or to proceed directly to caesarean section. Internal podalic version has the advantage of being quicker than caesarean section, particularly if an effective epidural is already in situ. If an epidural is not in situ, the woman can be transferred to theatre and a spinal or a general anaesthetic performed. If internal podalic version is successful, then caesarean section (with its attendant increase in maternal morbidity and implications for future deliveries) is avoided. The disadvantage is that a breech delivery is inevitable and rupturing the membranes can make subsequent caesarean section difficult. As the birth canal is already dilated and the second twin is usually smaller than the first, a breech delivery is still a safe option. Where maternal effort is poor (such as if a spinal anaesthetic is in situ), this is the one situation in which a breech extraction can be considered in experienced hands. Internal podalic version should be avoided if there is little liquor or with previous caesarean section, as there is increased risk of trauma to mother and fetus.

Caesarean section for transverse lie with reduced liquor is a difficult procedure and should be undertaken only by an experienced obstetrician. A low vertical, or even a classical, caesarean section should be considered, particularly in a preterm pregnancy. If there is difficulty with a delivery following a transverse lower uterine incision, it can be converted to a J incision.

Comments
This question tests your ability to handle an obstetric emergency safely. If you write something that is considered to be unsafe practice, the examiner may be allowed to use his discretion and fail you outright on the question.

So:

- If mentioning breech extraction, make it quite clear that the delivery of a second twin is only one of two instances in which this is justifiable in modern obstetric practice. The other is in delivery of a dead fetus.
- Point out that you recognise that a caesarean section with a transverse lie and no liquor can be extremely difficult and an experienced pair of hands is a prerequisite.

Suggested reading
Chamberlain G (ed) 1995 Turnbull's obstetrics. Churchill Livingstone, Edinburgh
James D K, Steer P J, Weiner C P, Gonik B (eds) 1994 High risk pregnancy – management options. Saunders, London
Local labour ward protocol

4. **A 38-year-old primigravid woman suffers from familial hyperlipidaemia and angina. She presents at 30 weeks' gestation with a singleton pregnancy, in early labour. Discuss optimal intrapartum management.**

Safe management of a patient with this uncommon problem requires the rapid involvement of experienced paediatricians, physicians and anaesthetists, in addition to senior obstetricians.

The woman should have an obstetric and a cardiorespiratory assessment, commencing with a review of the medical records and a full history and examination. The presence of heart failure, the fetal presentation, the presence of the fetal heartbeat and the progress in labour are of particular importance. The woman should have a baseline 12-lead electrocardiograph (ECG) and be commenced on cardiac and blood pressure monitoring and pulse oximetry. A prompt decision must be made as to whether or not labour should be stopped. It is usual to allow labour to continue in these circumstances, as often it is felt that continuation of the pregnancy poses a greater risk to the mother. Tocolysis using beta adrenoceptor agonists is inadvisable as it can precipitate heart failure. Nitrate medication itself has been used as a tocolytic but is relatively ineffective. Steroids would be given to induce surfactant production.

In the absence of an obstetric indication for caesarean section, a vaginal delivery is preferable in view of the lower maternal risk. If labour is established, intravenous access should be secured and a full blood count, urea and electrolytes, blood grouping and saving of serum requested. ECG, pulse oximetry and cardiotocography (CTG) should be continued. A partogram and an accurate fluid balance record must be kept. A midwife should be allocated to care for her exclusively in labour. The woman must take her normal medication during labour and nitrate medication must be available. An epidural is advisable. A 15 degree lateral tilt must be maintained if the woman is supine and lithotomy avoided if there are signs of heart failure. An elective forceps delivery may be considered to minimise maternal effort. The ventouse should not be used at this gestation.

The rapid increase in circulating volume following the third stage can precipitate heart failure or cardiac ischaemia, so ergometrine is contraindicated. A physiological third stage can also lead to cardiac compromise due to the increased risk of postpartum haemorrhage. Syntocinon can be used to minimise these risks.

Comments

This question, by its phrasing, excludes discussion of the antenatal and postnatal period.

In a case of an intercurrent medical illness, it is important to emphasise the importance of multidisciplinary input.

'Safe doctor' points:

- Ritodrine and ergometrine are contraindicated in cardiac disease.
- Elective forceps delivery is no longer performed for prematurity, but in this case it should be made clear that it may be indicated because of the maternal cardiac condition. The ventouse should be avoided under 32 weeks' gestation.

Suggested reading

Chamberlain G (ed) 1995 Turnbull's obstetrics. Churchill Livingstone, Edinburgh

James D K, Steer P J, Weiner C P, Gonik B (eds) 1994 High risk pregnancy – management options. Saunders, London

5. **Following a prolonged first labour and instrumental delivery, a 30-year-old woman continues to trickle blood per vaginum. Outline your management plan.**

As in all cases of postpartum haemorrhage, assessment of the haemodynamic status of the patient should take first priority. In this situation, a steady loss of blood can be underestimated, leading to sudden decompensation and onset of shock. Intravenous access must be secured and bloods should be taken for a full blood count (and compared with antenatal records), a clotting screen in case of insidious consumptive coagulopathy and a sample sent to blood transfusion in case blood needs to be cross-matched. Resuscitation with colloid solution and cross-matched blood would be appropriate in the shocked patient.

In this case, the most likely possibilities are that of genital tract trauma secondary to the instrumental delivery or an atonic uterus secondary to the prolonged labour. If the placenta appears incomplete, the patient must be taken to theatre for evacuation of the retained placental tissue. If the uterus feels poorly contracted, Syntometrine (ergometrine and oxytocin) or prostaglandin $F_{2\alpha}$ may be given. Any coagulopathy should be corrected with fresh frozen plasma. Involvement of senior colleagues and anaesthetists should be considered at this stage. Should these measures fail, the patient should be taken to theatre and under good anaesthesia (general anaesthesia or regional anaesthesia), the genital tract explored. The vulva and clitoris must be carefully examined. Particular care should be taken to search for the spiral tear classically associated with a rotational forceps delivery and also for a cervical tear. Rupture of the uterus would be rare in a primigravid woman, but the cavity of the uterus should nevertheless be checked for this, in addition to retained placental tissue. Bleeding from the apex of the episiotomy repair can also be deceiving. If the cause of the bleeding is not evident, the coagulation should be rechecked and consideration given to further prostaglandin administration. Should this fail, laparotomy followed by ligation of the anterior division of the internal iliac arteries or hysterectomy may be required. Care must be taken not to leave these measures too late. Haemorrhage remains one of the leading causes of maternal mortality.

Comments

The question said *outline*, therefore do not go into immense detail. 'The cervix must be inspected to exclude a cervical tear', rather than a detailed account: 'I would use two pairs of sponge forceps. The first I would place on the anterior lip of the cervix etc.'.

Mentioning the importance of haemorrhage regarding maternal mortality is a must in any question on this topic.

'Safe doctor' point.   In any question regarding haemorrhage or a collapsed patient, discuss resuscitation first. What would you tell *your* SHO to do first?

Suggested reading

Chamberlain G (ed) 1995 Turnbull's obstetrics. Churchill Livingstone, Edinburgh

Gilbert L, Porter W, Brown V A 1987 Postpartum haemorrhage: a continuing problem. British Medical Journal 94: 67–71

Glazener C M A, Abdalla M, Stroud P et al 1995 Postnatal maternal morbidity: extent, causes, prevention and treatment. British Medical Journal 102: 282–287

Hibbard B M, Anderson M A, Drife J O et al 1996 Report on confidential enquiries into maternal deaths in the United Kingdom 1991–1993. (Triennial series) HMSO, London

PAPER 2

1. Critically evaluate antenatal booking investigations.

The primary aim of these investigations is to detect conditions in which early detection allows intervention for the benefit of both mother and fetus. Adequate counselling is essential or the result can be unnecessary anxiety and a poor rapport between the woman and hospital.

Only a small number of women have iron deficiency anaemia at booking, but a full blood count is of low cost and can be justified as a baseline investigation. In the UK, the incidence of haemoglobinopathies is low, so haemoglobin electrophoresis can only be justified in certain ethnic groups. Blood group typing and antibody screens are essential to detect antibodies that could cross the placenta, to allow rapid cross-matching later in pregnancy and anti-D prophylaxis in rhesus-negative women. Rubella screening and puerperal vaccination has made a large impact in the past on the number of pregnancies affected. Rubella immunisation of children has greatly reduced the incidence of the wild infection. As the vaccination for non-immune mothers can only be offered postpartum, women could alternatively be screened at this time.

Syphilis and phenylketonuria are rare, but as early detection and prompt treatment avoid adverse effects in the fetus, screening is still cost-effective. The argument for screening at booking for hepatitis B, human immunodeficiency virus (HIV) and toxoplasmosis is growing. Knowledge of maternal HIV status allows the risk of vertical transmission to be reduced by the use of anti-retroviral drugs and the avoidance of breastfeeding.

Screening for asymptomatic bacteriuria is important, as this condition indicates a high risk for urinary tract infection. Routine ultrasound scan examination is of value in picking up non-viable pregnancies and multiple pregnancies, excluding pathology such as hydatidiform mole and allowing assessment of gestational age. If ultrasound assessment of gestational age is not required, detection of the fetal heart on Sonicaid confirms a viable pregnancy, and ultrasound scan examination can then be performed later in pregnancy to screen for anomalies. At present, genetic screening is considered to be a prenatal investigation, but with the advent of single gene therapy there may be a move to include these tests as booking investigations.

Comments
The importance of counselling can be mentioned in any question regarding antenatal screening.

Your answer must demonstrate your understanding of cost/benefit analysis. Discuss the rationale behind the screening programme in your hospital with your colleagues.

Did you start with this question? Remember to start with the question that you find the easiest.

Suggested reading
Chamberlain G (ed) 1995 Turnbull's obstetrics. Churchill Livingstone, Edinburgh

Enkin M, Kierse M J N C 1989 Vol 1: Pregnancy. In: Chalmers I (ed) Effective care in pregnancy and childbirth. Oxford University Press, Oxford

Pearson V 1994 Antenatal ultrasound screening. Health Care Evaluation Unit, University of Bristol, Bristol

Royal College of Obstetricians and Gynaecologists 1995 Report of Joint Working Group on Organisational Standards for Maternity Services. RCOG, London

2. A 22-year-old unbooked African woman presents at 24 weeks' gestation with abdominal pain. How would you reach a diagnosis?

As this woman is unbooked, a careful history assumes even greater importance. The woman should be asked regarding presenting and associated symptoms and the pregnancy. In addition, enquiries should be made in regard to recent foreign travel and whether or not she has a history of sickle cell anaemia. A full general examination should be performed, in particular to determine the site of the pain and, if there is a suspicion of premature labour, a vaginal examination performed. In the case of possible ruptured membranes, only a sterile speculum examination is performed. The differential diagnoses can be divided into those causes related to the pregnancy and those incidental to the pregnancy. Obstetric causes would include an abruption, premature labour, chorioamnionitis secondary to ruptured membranes, or polyhydramnios secondary to a twin pregnancy. Uterine fibroids are common in this ethnic group and can present in this way owing to acute (red) degeneration in pregnancy. Non-obstetric causes could be a torted ovarian cyst, urological (urinary tract infection or calculae), or a surgical cause such as appendicitis or cholecystitis. Medical disorders such as sickle cell crisis or gastroenteritis should not be forgotten. Assistance from surgical and medical colleagues should be sought as required.

Full booking investigations are important, including haemoglobin electrophoresis, white cell count and blood grouping. A Kleihauer test is indicated if a placental abruption is suspected, whereas urea and electrolytes, liver function tests and amylase are indicated if surgical pathology is suspected. A urine sample must be taken for culture and sensitivity to exclude a urinary tract infection. Ultrasound scan examination would be central to any investigations, both to investigate fetal well-being and to exclude twin pregnancy and/or polyhydramnios. However, ultrasound examination is unlikely to help with the diagnosis of placental abruption. In addition, the renal tract and gall bladder may also be investigated with ultrasound, or a plain radiograph may be taken. Contrast studies are inadvisable in pregnancy.

Comments
Did you stray outside the focus of this question: reaching a diagnosis?

It is important when answering this type of question to be tuned into the clues in the question. In this case, the specific ethnic group is given, which makes the mention of sickle cell disease/trait and uterine fibroids a must. As this crosses the boundaries diagnostically, multidisciplinary input is essential.

Suggested reading

Barron W 1984 The pregnant surgical patient: medical evaluation and management. Annals of Internal Medicine 101: 683

Chamberlain G (ed) 1995 Turnbull's obstetrics. Churchill Livingstone, Edinburgh

Enkin M, Kierse M J N C 1989 Vol 1: Pregnancy. In: Chalmers I (ed) Effective care in pregnancy and childbirth. Oxford University Press, Oxford

3. **After a normal vertex delivery of a healthy full-term infant, the woman collapses. How would you manage this obstetric problem?**

The first priority in such a case would be to institute basic resuscitation techniques. The woman should be placed flat and the airway, breathing and circulation checked. Simple syncope will rapidly show signs of recovery. Should a cardiac arrest have occurred, the medical team should be called and full resuscitation measures instituted. Otherwise, oxygen should be administered and intravenous access obtained. Baseline blood tests can be taken for full blood count, urea and electrolytes, a sample for cross-matching and a clotting screen should also be considered. Further management would depend on the working differential diagnosis. A history from midwife and patient (if high enough level of consciousness) and examination may be significant. The association of a fit, high blood pressure and preceding symptoms such as epigastric pain, headache or visual disturbance would suggest eclampsia. In these circumstances, reduction of the blood pressure and administering an anticonvulsant (such as diazepam) intravenously would be the next priority. A low blood pressure and palpation of the uterus per abdomen and the assessment of vaginal loss may indicate the cause to be hypovolaemic shock, indicating the need for rapid volume replacement, initially with colloid and then cross-matched or even group-specific or O-negative blood. If epidural anaesthesia is in situ, toxicity of local anaesthesia or a high-level block is a possibility, particularly if a 'top up' has been given shortly beforehand. An anaesthetic opinion should be sought. Preceding chest pain, palpitations or shortness of breath would indicate other possibilities. These would include a myocardial infarction, a pulmonary venous thromboembolism, a cardiac arrhythmia, or an amniotic fluid embolism. Following a 12-lead electrocardiograph, urgent chest X-ray and arterial blood gases, pulse oximetry and cardiac monitoring should be instituted. A medical opinion and that of the anaesthetic team is helpful, as transfer to the intensive care or coronary care unit would be appropriate in these conditions. Myocardial infarction has a high mortality risk of 35–45% in this group and the diagnosis is difficult, as the cardiac enzymes are often deranged after delivery. If in doubt, a radionuclide scan will demonstrate the damaged myocardium.

Comments

This is a 'safe doctor' question. The examiner is interested to read your logical approach to swiftly stabilising the maternal condition. *Always* discuss resuscitation *first*.

This is another question where it is important to mention the involvement of clinicians from appropriate specialities. Just because you have mentioned it in one question does not mean that you should omit it from the next! There is a different examiner for each question.

Suggested reading
Chamberlain G (ed) 1995 Turnbull's obstetrics. Churchill Livingstone, Edinburgh
Enkin M, Kierse M J N C 1989 Vol 1: Pregnancy. In: Chalmers I (ed) Effective care in pregnancy and childbirth. Oxford University Press, Oxford
Robson S C, Boys R J, Hunter S, Dunlop W 1989 Maternal haemodynamics after normal delivery and delivery complicated by postpartum haemorrhage. Obstetrics and Gynaecology 74: 234–239
Rosevear S K, Stirrat G M 1996 Handbook of obstetric management. Blackwell Science, Oxford

4. A primigravida presents at 32 weeks' gestation with confirmed spontaneous rupture of membranes (SROM). Justify your management.

The first priority is a clinical assessment of the woman by history and examination. Detection of other complicating factors such as the coexistence of a multiple pregnancy or pre-eclampsia is important. Essential information includes the time of membrane rupture, the nature of the vaginal loss, uterine activity and abdominal pain. On examination, a maternal and fetal tachycardia, pyrexia and uterine tenderness would indicate chorioamnionitis. Abdominal examination is important to assess fetal presentation and uterine activity, particularly in regard to possible premature labour. A sterile speculum examination will confirm membrane rupture, demonstrate any significant cervical dilatation and exclude a cord prolapse. A high vaginal swab (HVS) identifies potential pathogens such as group B haemolytic streptococcus. A digital examination is avoided unless the woman is established in labour, because of the presumed risk of introducing infection. A cardiotocograph is indicated to monitor the uterine activity and the condition of the fetus. The options for further management lie between conservative and active management. In the majority of centres in the United Kingdom, the attendant excess neonatal morbidity and mortality from a delivery at 32 weeks is felt to favour the conservative approach, whereas at 34 weeks' gestation, delivery is advocated. In the absence of any complicating factors and following discussion with the paediatricians, this case would be managed conservatively. The majority of her subsequent care would be as an inpatient, as intervening chorioamnionitis requires prompt delivery. Weekly HVSs would be taken to screen for vaginal pathogens. A rise in white cell count (or C-reactive protein) may give an early indication of intervening infection. An ultrasound scan examination will reveal the presentation and give further details of the fetal condition. Steroids should be given to improve fetal surfactant production, as they do not appear to mask infection as was originally feared. The place of prophylactic antibiotics has not been proven as yet. As the onset of premature labour is usually secondary to chorioamnionitis, tocolysis is avoided, except in the 48 hours after steroid administration, to allow fetal surfactant production to occur.

At 34 weeks, delivery would be considered, owing to the improved neonatal outlook.

Comments
This question says 'confirmed', therefore no marks will be given for diagnostic methods.

The key word in the question is *justify*. It is not enough to give a list of actions: the reason for each management point must be given.

A good examination technique is to look for the omissions in the question. This question does not say that there are no other complications which may influence management, e.g. multiple pregnancy etc.

Keep up to date with the progress of ORACLE.

Suggested reading
Cararach V, Botet F, Sentis J et al 1993 The maternal and perinatal consequences of premature rupture of membranes. Contemporary Review of Obstetrics and Gynaecology 5: 85–89

Chamberlain G (ed) 1995 Turnbull's obstetrics. Churchill Livingstone, Edinburgh

Duff P 1991 Premature rupture of membranes. Clinical Obstetrics and Gynaecology 34: 683–795

Enkin M, Kierse M J N C 1989 Vol 1: Pregnancy. In: Chalmers I (ed) Effective care in pregnancy and childbirth. Oxford University Press, Oxford

Wennstrom K D, Weiner C P 1992 Premature rupture of membranes. Clinical American 19: 247–401

5. **Following an uneventful pregnancy, a primigravid woman presents at 42 weeks' gestation. Compare and contrast the management options available.**

The management options lie between conservative management and active management, i.e. delivery after verifying that the calculated gestation is correct. The presence of a multiple pregnancy, pre-eclampsia, abnormal lie or presentation, or other complication, would obviously result in an increased likelihood of intervention and would also increase the chance of a caesarean section being the chosen method of delivery. Active management is the preferred option currently by many pregnant women and obstetricians. The obstetric advantage of induction of labour is that the increasing problem of placental insufficiency that occurs post-term is avoided. At 42 weeks' gestation, induction results in a decreased incidence of meconium and operative delivery in comparison to those pregnancies that are left until later intervention or the onset of spontaneous labour. On the other hand, some women do not find induction of labour acceptable. The traditional approach of 'sweeping the membranes' has been proven to increase the likelihood of labour intervening and is accepted by some. In the remainder, expectant management is considered safe, provided that there is no clinical evidence of fetal compromise. The fetus may be assessed by biometric measurement, biophysical assessment and Doppler ultrasound, as well as cardiotocography. A reasonable chance of vaginal delivery can still be anticipated. The method selected for induction of labour is dependent on the Bishop score of the cervix, which attempts to describe objectively how favourable the cervix is regarding induction. If the cervix is unfavourable, the use of prostaglandin E_2 prior to artificial rupture of the membranes and intravenous oxytocin has led to an improved vaginal delivery rate. In the future, mifepristone may be used in addition, as the available evidence suggests that this would lead to an improved outcome in cases of an unfavourable cervix.

Comments
This question covers an important area of uncertainty in obstetrics, where the policy radically alters with time and location!

There are several areas in obstetrics where there is more than one option available for management. This question demonstrates how your examination preparation should include familiarisation with the current school of thought and the importance of making up your own mind in advance of the examination!

Take this completed paper and ask someone to check your handwriting for legibility. It doesn't matter how good your answer is if no-one can read it!

Suggested reading
Chamberlain G (ed) 1995 Turnbull's obstetrics. Churchill Livingstone, Edinburgh

Hannah M E, Hannah W J, Hellmann J, Hewson S, Milner R, Willan A 1992 A Canadian multicentre post-term pregnancy group trial. Induction of labour as compared to serial antenatal monitoring in post-term pregnancy. A randomised controlled trial. New England Journal of Medicine 326: 1587–1592

Pitkin R M, Scott J R, Phelan J P (eds) 1989 Postdatism. Clinical Obstetrics and Gynaecology 32: 219–303

PAPER 3

1. Caesarean section can be justified on maternal request alone. Debate this statement.

There has recently been much discussion in the United Kingdom (UK) regarding this issue. In the United States of America, the increasing caesarean section rate has been partially attributed to increased patient choice in 'consumer-led' health care and significant medicolegal pressures. There has been concern that this pattern may be repeating itself in the UK. There is, however, a case for caesarean section on demand. This approach fits with the current philosophy of empowerment of women regarding birth choices. Women's concerns regarding labour and delivery and the potential long-term consequences cannot be ignored. Careful counselling can often allay these fears. Nevertheless, elective caesarean section largely avoids the risk of pelvic floor damage and its effect on continence, sexual function and the increased risk of prolapse. A normal vaginal delivery carries the lowest risk for mother and a non-compromised fetus, but a normal delivery can never be guaranteed. An elective caesarean section avoids the potential trauma to mother and fetus of an instrumental delivery and the higher maternal risk associated with an emergency caesarean section. In the absence of a recurrent obstetric indication, those who have had a previous caesarean section still have a good chance of subsequent normal vaginal deliveries.

The case against caesarean section on demand is based not only on the increased demand on limited resources, but also on the attendant increased risk of caesarean section in comparison to normal delivery. The maternal risks include the associated risks of haemorrhage, anaesthesia and thromboembolic disease. Thromboembolism is currently one of the leading causes of maternal mortality. The increased morbidity associated with the more minor problems such as wound infection must also be considered. The increased likelihood of repeat caesarean section in future pregnancies is also important. Not only is transient tachypnoea of the newborn more common in babies delivered by caesarean section, but in this situation there is an increased risk of surfactant deficiency if the caesarean section is performed at 38 weeks' gestation rather than awaiting the onset of spontaneous labour. In conclusion, a request for caesarean section must be considered carefully. A decision should be made only after thorough counselling of the patient and her partner.

Comments
Your answer should include a sensible risk/benefit analysis, including cost implications. The importance of accurate counselling of the woman and her partner must be stressed.

Central to your answer is an understanding of how an increase in maternal requests fits into the current picture of an increasing caesarean section rate.

This is a very topical question and has been a subject for much discussion in both the medical and the lay press.

sted reading

...on G M, Lomas J 1984 Determinants of the increasing caesarean birth rate. Ontario data 1979–1982. New England Journal of Medicine 311: 887–892

Borthen I, Lossins P, Skjaerven R et al 1989 Changes in frequency and indication for caesarean section in Norway, 1967–1984. Acta Obstetrica et Gynecologica Scandinavica 68: 589–593

Lomas J, Anderson G M, Domnick-Pierre K et al 1989 Do practice guidelines guide practice? New England Journal of Medicine 321: 1306–1311

2. **A 32-year-old parous woman presents at the booking clinic with a history of severe postnatal depression after her last delivery. Outline your approach to her care.**

This woman must be considered to be at high risk of developing postnatal depression following the current pregnancy, as a previous episode is an important risk factor. The initial approach should be to assess the woman's current status. The occurrence of depression antenatally indicates a high chance of severe depression postnatally, particularly if it occurs in the last trimester. A history of depressed mood, excessive anxiety, initial insomnia, early morning wakening, decreased libido and ideas of decreased self-worth, self-blame and guilt are all symptoms characteristic of depression. Stressful life events are also important risk factors, such as chronic marital or social difficulties or ambivalence about the pregnancy. Ideal management would include antenatal referral to a psychiatrist with a special interest in this field. Assessment by a clinical psychologist is also of value. Arrangements can then be made by the hospital psychiatric and community-based teams to follow up this woman postnatally. Direct access to services by the woman should be made available.

The primary care team should also be closely involved and kept informed. Careful antenatal preparation and increased support by the midwifery staff postnatally is valuable. There is evidence that breastfeeding is very important as it increases the woman's self-esteem. Postnatally, early discharge should be avoided and in severe depression, transfer to the mother and baby unit is required. Prophylactic treatment with progesterone or antidepressants has been tried with varying success and can be considered. Long-term follow-up must be performed as the peak incidence is at 6–12 weeks postnatally. Additional symptoms postnatally include worries regarding criticism from health service professionals and fears that they will take the baby away, excessive concern regarding a normal baby and preoccupation with feeding, or at the other end, failure to thrive of a baby.

The effects of postnatal depression can be severe and disabling and have major implications for child and family. As there is often no insight by the woman, the diagnosis of depression can be delayed. A multidisciplinary approach, involving vigilance and prompt action by both hospital and community-based teams, is essential.

Comments
The postnatal period is an area often neglected in busy revision schedules! However, in a balanced obstetrics paper, you are just as likely to get a postnatal question as a preconceptual or antenatal question.
Your answer must highlight the importance of good communication with the primary health care team.
In any condition involving long-term maternal morbidity, it is good to demonstrate your awareness of the social implications, particularly regarding child welfare.

Suggested reading
Cox J L, Connor Y, Kendell R E 1982 Prospective study of psychiatric disorders of childbirth. British Journal of Psychiatry 140: 111–117
Elliott S A 1989 Psychological strategies in the prevention and treatment of postnatal depression. Psychological aspects of obstetrics and gynaecology. In: Baillière's Clinical Obstetrics and Gynaecology 3(4): 879–904
Pitt B 1968 Depression following childbirth. British Journal of Psychiatry 114: 1325–1335
Ruben P C 1987 Prescribing in pregnancy. British Medical Association, London

3. **Following an uneventful twin pregnancy, a routine ultrasound scan examination shows fetal death of one twin in utero. Justify your management.**

Management is primarily dependent on the gestation, but consideration of parental views is also important. Careful counselling is crucial. In the first trimester, the loss of one twin is a common event and it is likely that the second twin will survive. Even when the fetus that has died is expelled from the uterus, there are documented cases of the second twin surviving. Expectant management would involve monitoring of the pregnancy by checking of the fetal heart at regular intervals. If the fetal death occurs after the limit of viability, around 24 weeks' gestation, then the risk of continuing with the pregnancy must be carefully weighed against the risk of premature delivery. The focus must be on assessing the risk to the second twin. Ultrasound scan examination, umbilical Doppler measurements and, after 28 weeks' gestation, biophysical profile and cardiotocography can be used. The development and growth of the second twin and the zygosity of the pregnancy would influence management. A monochorionic placenta would indicate a raised risk of shared circulation, putting the surviving twin at particular risk. The development of a coagulopathy is usually of slow onset, but monitoring of platelet assay and clotting studies is required. From 24 weeks' gestation, the fetus would require ultrasound biometry fortnightly and prophylactic steroids should be given to promote surfactant production. If premature labour occurs, no attempt is made to stop labour as this is likely to be a sign of fetal compromise. After 34 weeks' gestation, the risk of premature delivery is less than the risk of continuing with the pregnancy and therefore delivery would be expedited. As neonatal care improves, earlier delivery may be contemplated following discussion with the paediatricians. The mode of delivery should be the least traumatic for the surviving twin. The presence of a breech presentation, signs of compromise of the surviving twin or an unfavourable cervix would all suggest that caesarean section should be the method of choice. The intrauterine insult of this event results in a higher incidence of cerebral palsy, even if the fetus is not delivered prematurely, therefore careful paediatric surveillance is justified.

Comments
The omission of the gestational age from the question is actually the key to answering this question.
Build your answer step by step on different scenarios according to the gestational age. This logical approach is important, so that the examiner can easily follow your train of thought.
In any discussion of delivery, remember to include *timing* and *mode*.

Suggested reading
Chamberlain G (ed) 1995 Turnbull's obstetrics. Churchill Livingstone, Edinburgh
Enkin M, Kierse M J N C 1989 Vol 1: Pregnancy. In: Chalmers I (ed) Effective care in pregnancy and childbirth. Oxford University Press, Oxford
MacGillivray I, Campbell D M, Thompson B (eds) 1988 Twinning and twins. Wiley, Chichester

4. **Describe the intrapartum complications that are associated with a diabetic pregnancy at 38 weeks' gestation and discuss possible methods of prevention.**

The St Vincent Declaration (WHO 1992) that women with diabetes should have a pregnancy outcome approximating to that of a non-diabetic women has not been achieved. The majority of complications, including intrapartum complications, of diabetes can be avoided by tight diabetic control preconceptually and during the antenatal period. Preconceptual counselling and preparation is essential for women with insulin-dependent diabetes (IDDM) and non-insulin-dependent diabetes. The presence of an effective screening programme to ensure the early detection of gestational diabetes is equally important. A multidisciplinary approach should be adopted, involving obstetricians, midwives, primary care team, physicians, diabetic nurses and dietitians. Consultant-led care and hospital confinement allows optimum diabetic control and early detection of complications. Serial ultrasound scan examination may detect macrosomia and polyhydramnios. The majority of intrapartum complications are secondary to these two conditions, for example malpresentation, cord prolapse, obstructed labour and shoulder dystocia. Induction of labour at 38 weeks, or elective caesarean section, can be considered to avoid the risks a macrosomic baby might bring. In those cases in which a vaginal delivery seems achievable, delivery must take place on the hospital unit with an experienced obstetrician on hand. An individualised regime for glucose control is ideally devised antenatally by the diabetic team. Alternatively, a comprehensive diabetic protocol should be incorporated in the labour ward protocol. An intravenous infusion should be started and insulin dosage should be guided by serial blood glucose estimation. This should reduce the incidence of intrapartum hypoglycaemia or hyperglycaemia. There is an increased chance of fetal distress and therefore continuous cardiotocography is justified. Early detection of cephalopelvic disproportion may be achieved by careful observation of the progress on the partogram. Active management of labour may improve the outcome for both fetus and mother, by shortening the duration of the labour. Instrumental deliveries should be avoided or undertaken circumspectly, with the thought of possible shoulder dystocia in mind. Likewise, early recourse to caesarean section and performance of an episiotomy should be considered in view of the possibility of shoulder dystocia in a macrosomic baby.

Comments

This is a good example of multidisciplinary care and the importance of intrapartum protocols.

The St Vincent Declaration can be trotted out in most obstetric diabetic questions.

Anyone with a sound clinical background should enjoy this question. This is a good opportunity to demonstrate your awareness of the intrapartum risks. The message implied in the question is that discussion of shoulder dystocia is a must.

Suggested reading

Cousins L 1987 Pregnancy complications among diabetic women: review 1965–1985. Obstetrics and Gynaecology Survey 42: 140–149

Gillmer M D G 1983 Diabetes in pregnancy. Medicine (International) 35: 1639–1640

Krans H M J, Porta M, Keen H (eds) 1992 Diabetes care and research in Europe: the St Vincent declaration action programme. WHO

Reece E A, Coustan D R 1988 Diabetes mellitus in pregnancy. Churchill Livingstone, New York

5. **A 39-year-old woman conceives following infertility treatment. A routine ultrasound at 16 weeks reveals a quadruplet pregnancy. How would you counsel her?**

Counselling would be based on a detailed assessment of the individual case by careful history taking, clinical examination and appropriate investigation. Both the woman and her partner should be involved. The options include non-intervention, termination of the pregnancy or selective termination. Parity, ease of conception, the nature of subfertility treatment and the couple's religious and moral stance will influence the couple's decision. With non-intervention, there is a high chance of the loss of all four fetuses. This is unlikely to be acceptable in a woman with a long history of primary infertility, especially as further conception in a woman of 39 with subfertility is unlikely. A woman who does have the responsibility of other children to care for may find the prospect of a long inpatient stay and the huge impact of multiple birth on the family unit equally unacceptable. This is particularly true if transfer to a distant unit is required because of inadequate neonatal facilities locally. Owing to the likelihood of a premature birth, the incidence of cerebral palsy and the other sequelae of extreme prematurity are significant. In spite of these points, this approach may fit with the couple's moral point of view. The second approach may be to terminate the pregnancy. A couple with secondary infertility may opt for termination of the pregnancy to minimise the impact on the rest of the family unit. The reduced chance of conception owing to maternal age must be discussed. The option of selective termination provides the best chance of a live baby. Reduction to a twin pregnancy with preferential termination of identical fetuses produces the best chance for the remaining babies. There is a risk of miscarriage following the procedure and an increased risk of cerebral palsy in the surviving babies, but overall the risks are much lower than those associated with no intervention. There can be mixed emotional reactions to this approach, as the couple may experience guilt and find it difficult to grieve in view of the ongoing pregnancy. In all cases, continued counselling must be made easily accessible to the couple.

Comments

In any counselling question, general points can be included. Conduction of counselling in privacy, inclusion of the partner (and other family members if appropriate) and involvement of midwife counsellors.

It is important to discuss all options available as the decision depends on the couple's circumstances. Do not approach the question with tunnel vision and just focus on the pros and cons of what you consider to be the best option. That is not what the question asked!

Suggested reading

Brown G, Dawe E 1980 Some aspects of triplet pregnancies in England and Wales 1971–1975. British Journal of Obstetrics and Gynaecology 34: 134–135

Dawe E 1978 Triplet pregnancy. British Journal of Obstetrics and Gynaecology 85: 505–509

Loucopoulos A, Jewelewicz R, Vande Wiele R L 1982 Multiple gestations. Acta Geneticae Medicae et Gemellologiae 31: 263–266

PAPER 4

1. Critically appraise the input of multidisciplinary clinics into obstetric care.

In recent years, the use of multidisciplinary clinics in obstetric care has expanded considerably. A particular example is the care of the diabetic woman in pregnancy. These clinics have allowed diabetic patients to be managed more effectively on an outpatient basis, reducing hospital visits and improving quality of care. The management of intercurrent medical illness in such a clinic allows the concentration of resources and continuity of care. Communication is facilitated between health professionals and joint decisions are more easily reached. Access to senior opinion is improved. Other examples include a joint clinic with the obstetric anaesthetist, to allow antenatal assessment of problems such as backache with regards to regional anaesthesia, or the haematologist for those with clotting disorders. Prenatal clinics allow accurate counselling, preconceptual preparation and timing of the pregnancy. Intrapartum plans can be produced, allowing appropriate intrapartum management of women by junior staff, when senior and specialist advice is not immediately available.

Establishment of multidisciplinary clinics is usually only feasible in the larger units or for common conditions such as diabetes. In some smaller district general hospitals, the reduced workload means that these clinics are not viable, as they are not cost-effective. The reduced availability of consultant staff in a smaller district hospital means that special sessions cannot be allocated and therefore management relies on liaison between the specialists involved on a more casual basis. Careful planning of multidisciplinary care is essential for it to be successful. If these clinics are held in the antenatal clinic, the patient may not be able to have routine specialist tests, as the equipment may not be readily accessible. Decreased junior involvement in the decision-making process and in routine antenatal care in these cases can affect both the quality of training and continuity of care during admissions to hospital.

Comments

The candidate must demonstrate awareness of the central concept behind multidisciplinary clinics: improved accessibility of quality care. This is only common sense!

This seems a daunting question initially. Remember, no-one will have specifically revised for this sort of question. A common-sense approach and a few minutes' careful thought and planning will result in a satisfactory and well-structured answer.

Resist waffling, get straight to the point. In a closed marking system, waffling just wastes time and may lose you discretionary points.

Suggested reading

Department of Health 1993 Changing childbirth. Report of the Expert Maternity Group. HMSO, London

Enkin M, Kierse M J N C 1989 Vol 1: Pregnancy. In: Chalmers I (ed) Effective care in pregnancy and childbirth. Oxford University Press, Oxford

RCOG 1995 Report of Joint Working Group on Organisational
    Standards for Maternity Services. RCOG, London

2. **Having recently returned from a holiday abroad, a woman presents
   at 28 weeks' gestation with a persistent pyrexia of unknown origin
   and abdominal pain. How would you reach a diagnosis?**

The underlying cause of the temperature and abdominal pain may be
associated with pregnancy or incidental to the pregnancy. If incidental, the
cause may be secondary to intra-abdominal pathology or a systemic
illness. A careful history and examination should be performed to elicit
localising symptoms or signs. A history of suspected rupture of the
membranes or an offensive discharge suggests underlying
chorioamnionitis. A sterile speculum examination and a tender uterus
would support this. Premature labour must be excluded. Though rare, red
degeneration of a uterine fibroid as a cause of abdominal pain and pyrexia
should not be forgotten. A history of nausea, vomiting and diarrhoea
suggests gastroenteritis. The history of foreign travel increases the
possibility of salmonellosis, campylobacter and amoebic dysentery. The
symptoms could also be related to a surgical cause such as cholecystitis,
pancreatitis or appendicitis. Coexisting nausea, dysuria, frequency of
micturition and loin pain suggest a urinary tract infection, common in
pregnant women. A renal calculus may also present in this way, although
haematuria and severe colicky loin to groin pain is more characteristic. A
detailed travel history and history of any malarial prophylaxis and
immunisations should be taken. Signs such as a rash, lymphadenopathy,
jaundice (in the absence of cholecystitis), throat or chest signs suggest
systemic illness. Dependent on the area of travel, there may be a
possibility of infectious hepatitis (hepatitis A is common), malaria and
typhoid fever. Malaria is the commonest cause of fever worldwide.
    Investigations must include a full blood count with differential white cell
count. In suspected malaria, thick and thin blood films are requested.
Urea, electrolytes, liver function tests and serum amylase may be
indicated, as is a viral screen where there is coexistent jaundice. An
infection screen is mandatory and includes microscopy and culture of a
midstream specimen of urine, a higher vaginal swab and blood cultures.
If indicated, stool microscopy and culture and throat swabs are
performed. An ultrasound scan examination may confirm decreased
liquor volume in the case of ruptured membranes. Other imaging, for
example of the gall bladder, may be indicated by the clinical findings.

Comments
The inclusion of such a question in the examination is not unlikely.
The awareness of the College that many candidates are from overseas
means that on occasions they will include questions requiring basic
knowledge of practice outside the UK. However, common things are
common. It is far more likely that this lady has a urinary tract infection
than malaria!

Suggested reading
Bell D R (ed) 1994 Lecture notes on tropical medicine, 4th edn.
    Blackwell Science, London

3. A woman was involved in a road traffic accident at 26 weeks' gestation. Discuss the obstetric contribution to her care.

Accurate assessment of injuries is essential, as the nature and extent of injuries incurred determines subsequent management. The obstetrician may be asked regarding the risk posed to the fetus of investigations, surgery and medication. The benefit to the mother must be balanced against the risk to the fetus, bearing in mind that fetal well-being is dependent on maternal well-being. At 26 weeks, organogenesis is complete. The fetus can be screened from most radiological investigations and the risk of plain abdominal X-ray films is proven to be low.

Contrast studies have not been fully evaluated and should be avoided if possible.

Obstetric assessment, by history, clinical and ultrasound scan examination, is required. The main risk is that of placental separation caused by direct trauma, a wrongly positioned seat belt or a deceleration injury. This can pose a major risk to mother and fetus and prompt delivery is required: at this gestation often by a classical caesarean section. As intra-abdominal pathology is possible, a vertical skin incision (which can be extended) is advisable, as is both obstetric and surgical involvement. If the bleeding is of a lesser degree, particularly if the fetal heartbeat is absent, induction of labour may present less maternal risk. In slight vaginal bleeding, conservative management is appropriate. Tocolytic cover is inadvisable due to the cardiovascular side-effects and the vasodilatory effect of beta adrenoceptor agonists, which can lead to an increase in bleeding.

In cardiac arrest, there is evidence that rapid caesarean section can improve maternal outcome if there is no response after 20 minutes. Where the mother has suffered severe brain injury and a permanent vegetative state has been diagnosed, delivery can be performed with the consent of the next of kin, when there is a reasonable chance of viability.

Those women who recover from their injuries may experience further problems towards term with weight-bearing activity. Women who have experienced pelvic fractures may have a contracted pelvis. This is one of the remaining indications for pelvimetry by X-ray, computerised tomography or magnetic resonance imaging. Elective caesarean section is indicated in a contracted pelvis or reduced hip mobility.

Comments

This question specifically asks for the obstetric contribution, so do not discuss the role of the other members of the multidisciplinary team.

The emphasis in your answer should be towards the mother's welfare first.

The management of this case obviously depends on the degree and nature of injuries, so structure your answer around different scenarios.

Suggested reading

Buchsbaum H J 1968 Accidental injury complicating pregnancy. American Journal of Obstetrics and Gynaecology 102: 752–769
Drost T F, Rosemurgy A S, Sherman H F et al 1990 Major trauma in pregnant women: maternal/fetal outcome. Journal of Trauma 30: 574–578

Griffiths M, Siddall-Allum J et al 1993 Road traffic accidents in pregnancy – the management and prevention of trauma. In: Studd J (ed) Progress in obstetrics and gynaecology. Churchill Livingstone, Edinburgh, vol 10, pp 87–99

4. **Following a prolonged labour, a 17-year-old primiparous patient delivers a healthy 4050 g baby vaginally and subsequently has a massive postpartum haemorrhage. Discuss the priorities in the management of this obstetric emergency.**

Immediate resuscitation should begin with the woman placed supine and oxygen therapy given. Two large-bore canulae should be inserted, a full blood count, clotting studies and sample for cross-matching obtained and fluid replacement started (usually with colloid solution). O-negative blood is rarely required, as group-specific blood is usually swiftly available and can be given whilst awaiting a full cross-match. Senior obstetric staff and the labour ward anaesthetist should be called. It is important to determine if the placenta was delivered intact, if the third stage was managed actively and the mode of delivery. If placental tissue is retained, an oxytocin infusion may be commenced prior to a prompt manual removal in theatre. If genital tract trauma is suspected, prompt examination in theatre, followed by careful repair, is essential. The risk of genital tract trauma is higher in an instrumental delivery, particularly if rotational forceps have been used.

Uterine atony is likely following a prolonged labour in a primigravid woman. Palpation of the abdomen will reveal a poorly contracted uterus. Massage of the uterus can sometimes stimulate uterine activity. Syntometrine (oxytocin and ergometrine) may be repeated, followed by prostaglandin $F_{2\alpha}$. In continued bleeding, an experienced obstetrician should perform an examination under anaesthetic to exclude unsuspected genital tract trauma or retained remnants of placenta.

Prostaglandin $F_{2\alpha}$ can be repeated intramuscularly, or given directly into the uterine muscle (transabdominally or transcervically).

A consumptive coagulopathy may compound the blood loss at this stage. The use of bimanual compression or packing of the uterus may produce enough time for correction of any clotting abnormality by fresh frozen plasma and platelet infusion. The next step would be that of laparotomy proceeding to ligation of the anterior divisions of the internal iliac arteries or hysterectomy. Despite the young age of this patient, it would be important not to delay proceeding to hysterectomy unnecessarily, as haemorrhage is one of the leading causes of maternal mortality and morbidity.

Comments

Resuscitation first!

It is very important to emphasise that senior input must be requested at an early stage. Remember that this was one of the recommendations of the RCOG report (1992) *Maternal Mortality – The Way Forward.*

The question omits the type of delivery on purpose. A discussion regarding the association of instrumental delivery and genital tract trauma is therefore indicated.

Suggested reading

Chamberlain G (ed) 1995 Turnbull's obstetrics. Churchill Livingstone, Edinburgh

Gilbert L, Porter W, Brown V A 1987 Postpartum haemorrhage: a continuing problem. British Medical Journal 94: 67–71

Glazener C M A, Abdalla M, Stroud P et al 1995 Postnatal maternal morbidity: extent, causes, prevention and treatment. British Medical Journal 102: 282–287

Hibbard B M, Anderson M A, Drife J O et al 1996 Report on confidential enquiries into maternal deaths in the United Kingdom 1991–1993. (Triennial series) HMSO, London

Patel N (ed) 1992 Maternal mortality – the way forward. RCOG, London

5. **A primigravida presents with an unexplained stillbirth at 37 weeks' gestation. Review the psychological aspects of her care.**

The psychological care of women who have experienced a stillbirth has been a neglected area until recent years. The impact of such an event not only produces significant psychiatric morbidity for the woman and her partner, but can also have a devastating effect on her marriage and family as a whole. Crucial to the care of a couple in these circumstances is the role of an experienced midwife during labour and delivery. The couple should be encouraged to view, handle and even dress the baby. Naming the baby, and the referral to the baby by its given name at all times by the attending staff, emphasises the importance of the baby as an individual. Photographs, foot and hand prints and other mementoes should be gathered for the parents. If the parents decline these, they should be stored in the notes so that they may be retrieved later if the parents wish. The establishment of long-term memories of the baby is an important aid to the normal grieving process. Appropriate clergy may provide additional support, and compliance with religious rituals helps the process of grieving. The involvement of other relatives, such as grandparents, allows the open recognition of this sad event. This helps to improve communication in the family and legitimises the expression of grief. After delivery, help with the documentation and funeral arrangements is required. The primary care team should be informed so that prompt involvement in her care can be effected. Long-term open access for family members to counselling is required, particularly at times such as the anniversary of the event. Support groups such as SANDS (Stillbirth and Neonatal Death Society) may prove valuable. Memorial services are conducted by some hospitals on a yearly basis and can also act to channel the grief reaction. The woman and her partner should be seen following delivery by senior medical staff to review the results of investigations and to answer any queries the couple may have. Vigilance of health professionals is important to detect deviations from the normal grieving process and allow appropriate psychiatric referral.

Comments

This question very specifically asks about the psychological aspects of her care and *not* medical management.

Bereavement counselling and 'breaking bad news' are considered to be important parts of your training. Remember this could also figure in the oral assessment examination.

If you found this question difficult to answer, gain some background knowledge by talking to senior midwives who have often been specifically trained in this sensitive area.

Suggested reading

American College of Obstetricians and Gynaecologists 1986 Diagnosis and management of fetal death. Bulletin No 98

Kochenour N K 1987 Management of fetal demise. Clinical Obstetrics and Gynaecology 30: 322

PAPER 5

1. Evaluate the role of maternal serum screening for Down syndrome.

Evaluation of a screening test should take place in accordance with the World Health Organization (WHO) 1968 guidelines. Down syndrome is common and constitutes a major health problem, the baby often being physically as well as mentally handicapped, requiring major gastrointestinal or cardiac surgery. Targeted amniocentesis in older and therefore higher-risk mothers does not significantly reduce Down syndrome births because the increased birth rate in younger mothers results in a higher number of Down syndrome babies in this age group. Down syndrome is well understood and it places a huge burden on the family. Amniocentesis is the proven diagnostic test, but there is a risk of miscarriage. There is no treatment for Down syndrome, though termination of pregnancy can be offered. In couples in whom this is unacceptable, screening is not justified. The well-established serum 'triple test' uses maternal age, human chorionic gonadotrophin (hCG), alpha-fetoprotein (AFP) and oestriol to calculate a numerical risk. Modifications are available to attempt to reduce the false positive and negative rate (beta subunit of hCG, urea-specific neutrophil alkaline phosphatase) or to screen at an earlier gestation (ultrasound measurement of nuchal skin thickness). Certain conditions which alter these parameters have not been taken into account (multiple pregnancy, threatened miscarriage). Counselling of patients regarding the numerical risk is essential, as some women find the result difficult to comprehend. Some women find a non-diagnostic test stressful. The psychological implications of these tests have not been fully evaluated. The 'triple test' is cost-effective only if amniocentesis is performed in accordance with the results of the triple test. In these circumstances, if performed only on those women who would have a termination of pregnancy, it is probably cost neutral. However, despite the availability of serum screening, many women over 37 years old elect to have amniocentesis based on age alone, leading to an overall increase in amniocentesis and therefore cost. Future development of a test in which the fetal cells can be extracted from maternal blood is underway, which would serve as both a non-invasive diagnostic test and a potential screening test.

Comments

This is a rapidly expanding field. Though this subject has come up recently, the continued clinical controversy around this topic means that it is likely to be included at some point in the MRCOG Part 2.

Get the most recent review article on this subject the month before the examination and make sure that you are up to date.

Did you discuss other methods of screening? As the question specifically said serum screening, this will have incurred a heavy time penalty and gained no points!

Suggested reading

RCOG 1993 Report of the RCOG Working Party on biochemical markers and the detection of Down's syndrome. RCOG Press: 11

Wald N J, Densem J W, Smith D, Klee G G 1994 Four marker serum screening for Down's syndrome. Prenatal diagnosis 14: 707–716

2. A 30-year-old woman is known to be HIV-positive and is now 14 weeks' pregnant. Review the implications of her serostatus for her obstetric care.

Unless the woman has received preconceptual counselling (the ideal), she is likely to present with a number of concerns. Careful counselling is therefore essential. Then, of course, there will be concern regarding the effect of her HIV status on the pregnancy and health of the child.

The risk of antenatal vertical transmission of HIV is significant at around 10–15%. There are also concerns regarding the effect of a pregnancy on the health of the mother, in particular the risk of deterioration of the condition into AIDS. There may be concern regarding the ability of the woman to care for a child long term when the prognosis is poor. Some women may opt for termination of the pregnancy. Antenatal care should be focused on minimising risk of vertical transmission. Recent evidence has shown that reduction of viral load using antiretroviral drugs (such as zidovudine) has a definite effect, reducing transmission by two-thirds. At this stage of pregnancy, organogenesis is complete and therefore the teratogenesis risk would be low. There is also evidence that delivery by caesarean section also decreases the risk and may be considered.

If vaginal delivery is contemplated, there is the suggestion that procedures involving scalp trauma such as ventouse delivery, fetal blood sampling or affixing of a scalp electrode may lead to increased transmission. Breastfeeding should be discouraged (in the Third World countries, breastfeeding would be advocated owing to the high infant mortality in artificially fed babies). The risk of deterioration to AIDS is low. The progress of the HIV infection can be monitored by the viral load and the T lymphocyte profile (CD4). Such patients require multidisciplinary input, particularly with genitourinary medicine. Care must be taken that, if required, additional social support is in place prior to discharge.

Whilst maintaining strict patient confidentiality, precautions must be taken regarding staff. Although the normal protocols should be adequate if strictly adhered to, there is evidence that measures such as double gloving and eye protection are also of value in the protection of staff from HIV transmission.

Comments

This is very much a question of global importance. Another related topic which has been debated recently is the inclusion of routine HIV screening at booking. Include this in your revision schedule!

It helps to think of this as a real patient presenting in your antenatal clinic. In this way, your answer will reflect your approach to the woman as a whole, rather than just a medical problem and you are less likely to omit important aspects such as counselling.

When considering any question regarding a medical condition in a pregnant woman, think about the risk of the condition to the pregnancy and fetus and think about the risk pregnancy may have for the disease progression and maternal health. Do not forget to mention the need for additional social support.

Suggested reading

Brettle R P, Raab G M, Ross A et al 1995 HIV infection in women: immunological markers and the influence of pregnancy. AIDS 9: 1177–1184

Chin J 1990 Epidemiology; current and future dimensions of the HIV/AIDS pandemic in women and children. Lancet 336: 221–224

Johnson F, Brettle R, MacCallum L et al 1990 Women's knowledge of their antibody state: its effect on their decision whether to continue their pregnancy. British Medical Journal 300: 23–24

3. **A 28-year-old nulliparous woman has long-standing insulin-dependent diabetes mellitus (IDDM) and is known to have renal impairment secondary to diabetic nephropathy. She states her wish to plan a family. How would you counsel her?**

It is important to involve both the woman and her partner. A joint approach involving both obstetricians and renal physicians is appropriate. As this woman has no children, then the desire to have children may well outweigh the risks associated with proceeding with a pregnancy. As the diabetic-related complications are likely to increase with time, the earlier the pregnancy occurs the better the outcome. The first consideration is the effect that pregnancy would have on diabetic-related complications. Patients usually require frequent upwards alterations of insulin during pregnancy. Poor control will lead to a rapid deterioration of diabetic retinopathy as well as nephropathy. An increase in hypoglycaemic and hyperglycaemic episodes can occur and inpatient management may be required to obtain the control necessary to decrease pregnancy complications. The added load of pregnancy can precipitate renal failure requiring dialysis and the deterioration may be permanent. The probable outcome of the pregnancy can be crudely assessed according to the current degree of renal impairment, according to the creatinine clearance values. Those women with a creatinine clearance of under 180 μmol/L have poorer pregnancy outcome. The other area that should be discussed is the possible effect on the fetus. The importance of tight diabetic control preconceptually and throughout pregnancy to decrease the risks of fetal abnormality and fetal macrosomia must be emphasised. The discussion should also cover the increased likelihood of preterm delivery secondary to maternal and fetal complications. If, following the full discussion, the decision is to proceed with trying for a pregnancy, general advice such as taking folic acid, stopping smoking and weight reduction in cases of obesity should be given. Plans should be made to optimise diabetic control and for the couple to continue to use contraception until the glycosylated haemoglobin (or fructosamine) is within an accepted range. Continued contact with the obstetric team is advisable, as a significant proportion of these women suffer with subfertility, particularly if there is a moderate to severe renal impairment.

Comments

Did you consider the effect of the diabetes on the pregnancy and vice versa?

As with all preconceptual questions, general advice should be given regarding folic acid etc (see Paper 6, Question 1).

Preconceptual advice for intercurrent medical conditions to contraceptive advice if decided against pregnancy.

Preconceptual advice for intercurrent medical conditions:

* General: folic acid, stop smoking, weight reduction, etc.
* Situation: partner involvement, multidisciplinary involvement
* Risk assessment: effect of condition on the pregnancy, effect of pregnancy on the condition
* Plan for pregnancy and mode of delivery: e.g. hospital confinement, pregnancy timing
* Contraceptive advice if decision is against pregnancy.

Suggested reading

Chamberlain G (ed) 1995 Turnbull's obstetrics. Churchill Livingstone, Edinburgh

Cousins L 1987 Pregnancy complications among diabetic women: review 1965–1985. Obstetrics and Gynaecology Survey 42: 140–149

Gillmer M D G 1983 Diabetes in pregnancy. Medicine (International) 35: 1639–1640

James D K, Steer P J, Weiner C P, Gonik B (eds) 1994 High risk pregnancy – management options. Saunders, London

4. A primigravida presents at term with a persistent occipitoposterior position and failure to progress in the second stage of labour. How would you select an appropriate method of delivery?

The options lie between awaiting a normal delivery and expediting delivery by an instrumental or operative delivery. If the woman has been in the active phase of the second stage of labour for a significant length of time and advancement has ceased despite adequate uterine activity, intervention is appropriate. Clinical assessment and examination of the partogram and cardiotocograph will determine the appropriate mode of delivery. Caesarean section is appropriate if there are signs of cephalopelvic disproportion. These include slow progress in the first stage of labour, short maternal stature, large baby and the presenting part more than one-fifth palpable per abdomen. Per vaginum examination may suggest a contracted pelvis or demonstrate the head stationed above the ischial spines, vulval oedema or significant moulding and caput. The fetal condition, as assessed by examination of the cardiotocograph and the colour of the liquor, may also influence the decision.

If the head is very low in the pelvis and there is little caput or moulding, then it may be appropriate to deliver without rotation by Neville-Barnes forceps or the ventouse. If the position of the head is midcavity and a rotational delivery contemplated, regional anaesthesia is advisable. With improved analgesia, a manual rotation to occipitoanterior position may be accomplished. If not, the options lie between the ventouse and a rotational forceps delivery. The ventouse has the advantage that it is associated with a much lower risk of maternal trauma. Provided the cup can be positioned on the vertex (a special Bird occipitoposterior cup is ideal), flexion of the head and autorotation occurs. Flexion of the head using forceps is more difficult and the risk of maternal trauma is higher. Although the incidence of scalp trauma is lower with a forceps delivery, there is no long-term difference in fetal outcome between the two techniques. The ventouse would therefore be the primary choice for vaginal delivery in this case. As the ventouse is a mechanical device, and therefore prone to equipment failure, a rotational forceps would be a safe alternative in experienced hands.

Comments

The hint is in the question. Although the examiner is looking for a discussion of forceps versus the ventouse, the phrasing 'appropriate mode of delivery' includes caesarean section and manual rotation also.

Remember the current recommendation that the ventouse be used as the primary method of instrumental delivery.

Remember the importance of the partogram in the assessment of possible CPD, as well as clinical examination.

Suggested reading

Chamberlain G (ed) 1995 Turnbull's obstetrics. Churchill Livingstone, Edinburgh

Enkin M, Kierse M J N C 1989 Vol 1: Pregnancy. In: Chalmers I (ed) Effective care in pregnancy and childbirth. Oxford University Press, Oxford

Gee H, Olah K S 1993 Failure to progress in labour. In: Studd J (ed) Progress in obstetrics and gynaecology. Churchill Livingstone, Edinburgh, vol 10, pp 159–181

Gleeson N C, Gormally S M, Morrison J J, O'Regan M 1992 Instrumental rotational delivery in primiparae. Irish Medical Journal 85: 139–141

5. **During an artificial rupture of membranes (ARM) at 8 cm cervical dilatation, sudden bleeding was associated with a profound fetal bradycardia. Give a detailed account of your management.**

The first priority would be to assess the status of the mother, regarding vital signs and degree of blood loss. The anaesthetist would be called. If there are signs of maternal shock, resuscitation should be instituted without delay, oxygen therapy started and the mother placed on her left side. Secure intravenous access should be obtained and intravenous fluids such as colloid given. Blood should be sent for a full blood count, clotting screen and blood grouping and blood cross-matched if required. Examination of the woman may suggest the underlying cause, for example abdominal pain would suggest placental abruption. The maternity notes may reveal a recent ultrasound scan report demonstrating the placental site. The most likely diagnosis would be that of a placental abruption or a placenta praevia (although this should have been noted during vaginal examination). Where the maternal status appears unaffected and the bleeding is slight, vasa praevia should be suspected. With all these causes, it is likely that the condition of the fetus will continue to deteriorate, as evidenced by continued cardiotocograph abnormality, and delivery must be expedited. The paediatricians must be informed. Prior to full dilatation, or with the coexistence of another complication such as a breech presentation or multiple birth, caesarean section would be the first choice. Rapid progression to full dilatation may occur. In these cases and also in some multigravidae, a ventouse may be attempted prior to full dilatation. There must be no evidence of cephalopelvic disproportion and the head must be at or below the ischial spines. The main determinant of fetal outcome with a persistent bradycardia is time interval to delivery and therefore an instrumental delivery may well be quicker than a caesarean section in these circumstances. The disadvantage of an instrumental delivery is that it is another stress on an already compromised fetus and therefore the predicted ease of vaginal delivery must be considered.

Comments
Resuscitation first.

Note the omission of parity in the question. In a parous woman, a ventouse could be contemplated. The coexistence of any other pathology is also omitted.

A high standard would be expected, as this question is testing your competence in handling a labour ward emergency.

Suggested reading
Chamberlain G (ed) 1995 Turnbull's obstetrics. Churchill Livingstone, Edinburgh
James D K, Steer P J, Weiner C P, Gonik B (eds) 1994 High risk pregnancy – management options. Saunders, London

PAPER 6

1. A 27-year-old renal transplant recipient is contemplating a pregnancy. How would you counsel her?

The counselling of this woman and her partner pivots on the accurate assessment of the risk to the woman relative to the chance of a successful pregnancy and therefore must involve the renal physicians. A successful outcome for both mother and baby is closely linked to the degree of renal impairment and the presence of any graft rejection at the time of conception. Favourable factors would include: good health 2 years following the transplant, no proteinuria or hypertension, a serum creatinine of less than 180 μmol/L and a low requirement of immunosuppressive drugs. If she has a significant degree of renal impairment, she may suffer from subfertility and be at higher risk of miscarriage. If she should conceive, she may well require renal dialysis owing to the extra demands of pregnancy. Although an improvement in renal function should be anticipated postnatally, the long-term effects on kidney function are uncertain. There is no evidence of an increased incidence of graft rejection in pregnancy but the diagnosis (clinical features, ultrasound and renal biopsy) and treatment can be difficult during pregnancy. The main risk to the pregnancy is that of deteriorating renal function culminating in a premature delivery, so strict compliance with and control of medication is essential. The teratogenicity of steroids, azathioprine and cyclosporin appears to be low.

General preconceptual advice regarding folic acid supplementation and early hospital booking for antenatal care is essential, as is the timing of such a pregnancy. It may be necessary to alter medication or await a suitable interval following transplant or episode of graft rejection. The probable pattern of antenatal care should be discussed, such as total consultant-led care with multidisciplinary input and possible requirements for inpatient admission. Renal transplant does not preclude a normal delivery, but caesarean section may be needed in those women with impaired skeletal development, or to effect a premature delivery, or if the fetal condition requires it.

The impact of a high-risk pregnancy on the family unit is significant. Some women (particularly multiparae) may decide against a further pregnancy. If the couple decide against a pregnancy, contraception must be discussed.

Comments

Consider this in two parts: first the effect of the pregnancy on the maternal condition and secondly the effect of the maternal condition on the pregnancy.

This is a preconceptual counselling question. See Paper 5, Question 3.

Suggested reading

Becker G J, Fairley K F, Whitworth J A 1985 Pregnancy exacerbates glomerular disease. American Journal of Kidney Disease 6: 266–272

Chamberlain G (ed) 1995 Turnbull's obstetrics. Churchill Livingstone, Edinburgh

James D K, Steer P J, Weiner C P, Gonik B (eds) 1994 High risk pregnancy – management options. Saunders, London

2. **A 23-year-old who had a forceps delivery is found to have had a third-degree tear. Give a detailed account of your management.**

An experienced obstetrician should perform a meticulous assessment of the genital tract trauma under regional or general anaesthesia. This would take place in the operating theatre with the woman in lithotomy position and with adequate lighting and assistance. Prior to this, informed consent must be obtained and a sample sent for grouping and saving of serum or cross-matching of blood, dependent on the attendant blood loss. Prophylactic antibiotics should be given to minimise infection. The vagina must be carefully examined for signs of other trauma. After a rotational forceps delivery, a deep spiral vaginal tear is characteristic. If exploration of the uterus or cervix is required, this should be performed prior to repair of the third-degree tear. The perineal tear must be examined to see if the damage is a partial- or full-thickness tear of the anal sphincter and if the rectal mucosa has been breached. Polyglycolic sutures are suitable as they are absorbable and cause minimal tissue reaction. The repair is started above the apex of the rectal mucosa, using two layers of fine polyglycolic sutures, everting the mucosal edges into the rectum. The vaginal mucosa is repaired with a continuous suture. Care must be taken to carefully identify the ends of the anal sphincter, as they often retract, and perform accurate apposition using interrupted or figure-of-eight sutures. An overlapping repair is preferable. The perineal muscle is repaired with interrupted sutures, and the skin with either subcutaneous or interrupted sutures. As a guide, the anus must accommodate a finger at the end of the procedure and the vagina two fingers. Adequate analgesia must be prescribed in addition to stool softeners to avoid constipation. The physiotherapist will initiate a programme of pelvic floor exercises.

Hospital review and prompt referral for specialist opinion is important in those women who develop faecal incontinence.

The risk of a repeat third-degree tear is not high if a normal vaginal delivery is achieved, but an elective episiotomy may be considered if the perineum appears rigid. Elective caesarean section should be performed in those who had further problems following the repair.

Comments
'Give a detailed account' would be an unusual question, as most topics are too broad to be covered in a short essay. However, if this question does occur, the topic is likely to be straightforward, examining knowledge that any labour ward registrar is expected to have. To score highly relatively to other candidates, a thorough and systematic approach is essential. Another topic in this category includes 'the management of shoulder dystocia'. Write an essay plan *now*!

Remember that this question is not confined to the actual repair. Points such as follow-up arrangements and the use of prophylactic antibiotics are also important.

Suggested reading
Chamberlain G (ed) 1995 Turnbull's obstetrics. Churchill Livingstone, Edinburgh
Enkin M, Kierse M J N C 1989 Vol 1: Pregnancy. In: Chalmers I (ed) Effective care in pregnancy and childbirth. Oxford University Press, Oxford
Rosevear S K, Stirrat G M 1996 Handbook of obstetric management. Blackwell Science, Oxford

3. **A successful amniocentesis of one of two gestation sacs shows that the chromosomal pattern is consistent with Edward's syndrome, while the other fetus has a normal karyotype. Critically discuss the management options.**

The management would hinge on careful counselling of the couple concerned. Counselling would be based on a detailed assessment of the individual case by careful history taking, clinical examination and appropriate investigation. The options include non-intervention, termination of the pregnancy or selective termination. Non-intervention may fit best with the couple's moral and religious views. The couple should be warned that the fetus with Edward's syndrome may not survive and be stillborn. This approach presents the least risk for the normal twin, although it is not devoid of risk. In the event of fetal death in utero, there is a risk of premature labour and delivery. The impact of such a birth on the family unit can be profound. Caring for a healthy twin at the same time as a baby with a shortened life span can be traumatic. The couple must receive ongoing counselling and support throughout pregnancy.

The couple may opt for termination of the pregnancy. A couple in whom the pregnancy was unplanned and who are ambivalent regarding the pregnancy may opt for this approach. The couple may feel unprepared to continue with a pregnancy that is complicated, despite the prospect of the loss of a normal baby. This approach not only avoids the delivery of a baby with Edward's syndrome, but also avoids the chance of a surviving child with the sequelae of extreme prematurity. Selective termination of the baby with Edward's syndrome is the chosen option in many cases. Although there is a risk of miscarriage and premature labour secondary to the procedure, the prospects for a healthy surviving baby are high. Mixed emotional reactions are common, as the couple may experience guilt and find it difficult to grieve in view of the ongoing pregnancy. Continued counselling and support must be made easily accessible to the couple. The couple can be reassured that the risk of recurrent chromosomal abnormality in further pregnancies remains low, provided parental karyotypes are normal.

Comments
The gestation is not stated in the question, nor are any other obstetric details. Obviously the gestation influences the management.

Junior obstetric staff often have limited experience in this field. As these cases tend to be counselled and managed exclusively by the senior obstetric staff, take time to discuss memorable cases that your consultant can recollect. Then read round the subject. The information is much more likely to stick in your memory.

Suggested reading

Chamberlain G (ed) 1995 Turnbull's obstetrics. Churchill Livingstone, Edinburgh

Enkin M, Kierse M J N C 1989 Vol 1: Pregnancy. In: Chalmers I (ed) Effective care in pregnancy and childbirth. Oxford University Press, Oxford

Simpson J, Golbus M, Martin A, Sarto G 1982 Genetics in obstetrics and gynaecology. Grune & Stratton, Orlando

4. **The labour ward statistics reveal that the caesarean section rate at your hospital has climbed over 5 years from 12% to 25%. How would you address this problem?**

The most difficult task would be to decide what is an appropriate rate for this unit. A doubling of the rate seems concerning, but may be due to a change in the workload of the unit. For example, upgrading of the neonatal unit to receive referrals from the rest of the region obviously would lead to an increase in the caesarean section rate. The increase in high-risk obstetric patients secondary to in utero transfers may entirely account for the increase. A comparison of the caesarean section rates between different consultants and with nearby hospitals with similar workloads may be helpful.

A careful audit of caesarean sections should be performed. This would include a study of the proportion of elective and emergency procedures, parity and gestation. If the increase seems to be attributable to increased elective caesarean sections, appropriate intervention may be devised. Conversion of a 'caesarean section for all breech presentations' policy to a selective policy is a possibility. If the increase appears to be due to repeat caesarean sections for non-recurrent causes, then allowing more to have a trial of labour is also an option. The increase in caesarean sections may be attributable to patient choice. Improved counselling and education of the couple, though time-consuming, may have a limited impact.

Production of a labour ward protocol addressing the active management of labour in primigravid women has been shown to have a dramatic impact in reducing the emergency caesarean section rate. Introduction of fetal blood sampling and greater input of senior staff has been shown to decrease the incidence of caesarean section for presumed fetal distress. A review of the induction policy may be appropriate, as the use of prostaglandins and an evidence-based approach to the selection of women for induction of labour can reduce the chance of caesarean section. Mifepristone cervical priming may also decrease the incidence of failed induction of labour.

The results of the audit should be openly discussed in the unit and guidelines governing caesarean section produced. Any interventions introduced should be the subject of further audit to close the audit loop.

Comments

This is essentially an audit question. Familiarise yourself with the audit cycle again.

The answer needs to demonstrate a logical approach to analysing the problem. This is a broad question asking for a large range of interventions dependent on the cause. Don't write an essay solely on the active management of labour!

Suggested reading

Anderson G M, Lomas J 1984 Determinants of the increasing caesarean birth rate. Ontario data 1979–1982. New England Journal of Medicine 311: 887–892

Borthen I, Lossins P, Skjaerven R et al 1989 Changes in frequency and indication for caesarean section in Norway, 1967–1984. Acta Obstetrica et Gynecologica Scandinavica 68: 589–593

Lomas J, Anderson G M, Domnick-Pierre K et al 1989 Do practice guidelines guide practice? New England Journal of Medicine 321: 1306–1311

Thiery M, Derom R 1986 Review of evaluation studies on caesarean section. Part 1: Trends in caesarean section and perinatal mortality. In: Kaminski M, Brent G, Beukens P et al (eds) Perinatal care delivery systems. Oxford Medical Publication, Oxford, pp 93–113

5. **Outline the management of a singleton small-for-dates pregnancy at 30 weeks' gestation for the remainder of the pregnancy.**

The gestation must be confirmed by calculation based on the last menstrual period and early ultrasound scan examinations. A small-for-dates pregnancy can be as a result of a constitutionally small baby or a growth-retarded baby. An ultrasound scan examination is very important. Asymmetrical growth, sparing of the head circumference or biparietal diameter with a decreased abdominal circumference, is more indicative of a growth-retarded baby, although early-onset growth retardation may be symmetrical. Measurements below the 10th centile are suspicious of growth retardation. A repeat anomaly screen should be performed as there is increased risk of fetal abnormality. Repeat biometry 2 weeks later may confirm growth retardation, as the growth in these cases deviates from the centile lines. In a growth-retarded fetus, assessment of the current fetal condition by biophysical profile, cardiotocograph and umbilical Doppler blood flow is important. Fetal acid–base measurement by cordocentesis is confined to specialist centres. The most important indicators are that of low liquor volume, abnormal cardiotocograph and absent or reversed end-diastolic flow on Doppler examination of the umbilical blood flow. If there is evidence of significant fetal compromise, delivery is required. Ideally, antenatal steroids should be administered to aid lung maturation and delivery timed for 48 hours later.

In a fetus in good condition, full assessment would be performed every 2 weeks and delivery effected if there were any sign of fetal compromise. The woman can be advised of the importance of fetal movements and repeat cardiotocography may be performed. At 34 weeks' gestation, the threshold for elective delivery drops because of the improved neonatal outcome. The timing of delivery will be made in consultation with the neonatologists and should occur when the risk of remaining in utero outweighs the risk of premature delivery. In growth retardation, the pregnancy should not be allowed to go past term, to avoid superadded placental insufficiency. There is a low threshold for caesarean section, the degree of fetal compromise, the presentation, the onset of spontaneous labour or ease of induction of labour being considered. Continuous fetal heart monitoring should be employed intrapartum.

Comments
'Outline' means giving a logical, step by step approach to management without concentrating in detail on the mechanics of any step.

Management includes clinical assessment, investigations and a plan for delivery (mode and timing).

Suggested reading

Brar H, Rutherford S 1988 Classification of intrauterine growth retardation. Seminars in Perinatology 12: 2–10

Campbell S 1977 Fetal growth. Clinical Obstetrics and Gynaecology 1: 41–65

Chamberlain G (ed) 1995 Turnbull's obstetrics. Churchill Livingstone, Edinburgh

James D K, Steer P J, Weiner C P, Gonik B (eds) 1994 High risk pregnancy – management options. Saunders, London

Sharp F, Fraser R B, Milner R D G (eds) 1989 Fetal growth. RCOG, London, p 313

Simpson G, Creasy R 1984 Obstetric management of the growth retarded baby. Clinical Obstetrics and Gynaecology 11: 481–497

PAPER 7

1. Compare and contrast the methods used in invasive prenatal diagnosis.

The commonest occasion on which invasive prenatal diagnosis is used is in the diagnosis of chromosomal abnormalities such as Down syndrome. The two most common techniques used are amniocentesis and chorionic villous sampling (CVS). Amniocentesis is a well-established technique and carries an excess risk of miscarriage of 0.5–1%, whereas CVS carries a higher risk of miscarriage of around 2%. However, CVS can be performed transabdominally, which carries a lower fetal loss rate and CVS has the advantage of being readily performed at an earlier gestation, typically 8–12 weeks' gestation, compared to 15–18 weeks for amniocentesis. When the procedure is being performed to screen for a condition in which termination of the pregnancy is a real possibility, early diagnosis is very important. In some centres, amniocentesis is being performed at a much earlier gestation, but it is thought to carry a higher risk. There has been some concern regarding misdiagnosis with CVS, due to the incidence of placental mosaicism (eight times more common than with amniocentesis). With both techniques, there have been questions raised regarding the long-term sequelae of the procedures. In CVS, there seems to be an increased incidence of fetal limb abnormalities, particularly when performed under 9 weeks' gestation. Amniocentesis has been variously linked to respiratory difficulties and postural deformities.

In certain conditions such as the haemoglobinopathies and in cases of viral infection, cordocentesis is required. This carries a higher fetal loss rate of up to 10%, mainly due to fetal exsanguination. This technique is a more difficult procedure, with a longer learning curve. The risk therefore varies markedly as it is operator dependent. Fetoscopy was used to visualise anatomical abnormalities and carried a significant risk. Its use has declined due to the improved resolution of ultrasound scan machines. Cordocentesis and fetoscopy should be confined to specialist centres.

Comments
Features that could be included are the appropriate timing of the test, speed of results, accuracy of the test (specificity and sensitivity), complication rate, acceptability to the woman.
    Did you concentrate on invasive tests?

Suggested reading
Rhoads G G 1989 The safety and efficacy of chorionic villus sampling for early prenatal diagnosis of cytogenetic abnormalities. New England Journal of Medicine 320: 609

Simpson N E, Dallaire L, Miller J R et al 1976 Prenatal diagnosis of genetic disease in Canada: report of collaborative study. Canadian Medical Association Journal 15: 739–748

2. **Following an uneventful singleton pregnancy, a woman presents at the antenatal clinic at 36 weeks' gestation. She has one other child born by caesarean section, owing to failure to progress in labour. Justify how you would reach a decision regarding her mode of delivery.**

Consideration of patient choice is essential when reaching a decision regarding the mode of delivery. Even in an unselected group of patients labouring following a previous caesarean section, around 80% will achieve a vaginal delivery. In the majority of cases, a carefully conducted trial of labour is a reasonable possibility. Repeat caesarean sections play an important part in the increasing caesarean section rate, so encouragement of women to undergo a trial of labour may reduce the caesarean section rate. This must be balanced against the fear many women have of a long protracted labour culminating in an inevitable emergency caesarean section. An increasing number of women are opting for the certainty of an elective caesarean section and an elective procedure carries a significantly lower maternal risk than an emergency procedure. An accurate assessment of the chances of achieving a vaginal delivery is essential to accurately counsel the woman and her partner.

The assessment should begin with analysis of the last labour, to determine if there is a recurrent cause for the non-progression of labour. Where necessary, and if time allows, records must be obtained from the previous hospital. The weight of the baby, the presentation, e.g. occipitoposterior, the use of Syntocinon and whether progress ceased in the first or second stage of labour is important information. The antenatal progress in the current pregnancy should be examined, as there may be a coincidental indication for caesarean section. An abnormal presentation, fetal compromise, multiple pregnancy, intercurrent illness or pre-eclampsia are examples. On examination, maternal short stature and a large baby on clinical estimation indicate a higher risk of cephalopelvic disproportion. Engagement of the fetal head is a favourable sign. If there is difficulty assessing fetal size or presentation, ultrasound scan examination can be performed. The traditional clinical assessment of the pelvic size during vaginal examination and X-ray pelvimetry are now considered to be poor indicators of outcome. They retain a place in some selected cases, such as pelvic deformity following pelvic fractures. Computerised tomography may have a place in the future, owing to superior accuracy in comparison to X-ray pelvimetry.

Comments
The examiner is obviously looking for the general concept that, even in a non-elective policy, a high proportion will achieve a vaginal delivery.

Don't forget to mention the importance of considering the woman's choice whenever discussing mode of delivery. The rest of the essay should be a concise account of the favourable and unfavourable factors for vaginal delivery and the appropriate methods of assessment.

X-ray pelvimetry is no longer considered to be of use in this type of assessment.

Suggested reading

Flamm B L 1985 Vaginal birth after caesarean section: controversies old and new. Obstetrics and Gynaecology 28: 735

Meehan F P, Rafla N M, Bolaji I I 1993 Delivery following previous caesarean section. In: Studd J (ed) Progress in obstetrics and gynaecology. Churchill Livingstone, Edinburgh, vol 10, pp 213–228

Meier P R, Porreco R P 1982 Trial of labour following caesarean section: a two year experience. American Journal of Obstetrics and Gynaecology 144: 671

Yetman T J, Nolan T E 1989 Vaginal birth after caesarean section: a reappraisal of risk. American Journal of Obstetrics and Gynaecology 161: 1119

3. **A primigravida with a multiple pregnancy attends for a routine antenatal visit at 34 weeks' gestation. Her blood pressure is found to be 160/100 mmHg and urinalysis reveals 2 g of protein. Justify your management.**

In view of the multiple pregnancy and primigravidity, this woman is at significant risk of pre-eclampsia and should be admitted for immediate assessment. Signs of a genuine pre-eclampsia include continuing proteinuria and hypertension (compared with the first trimester blood pressure recordings). Proteinuria may also be produced by contamination of the sample by vaginal discharge or by a urinary tract infection. A midstream specimen of urine (MSSU) must be sent for both microscopy and culture. Quantification of the proteinuria can be attempted by using a 24-hour urine measurement. Care must be taken that the correct size of blood pressure cuff is used and serial blood pressure measurement commenced. Other symptoms and signs of pre-eclampsia must be elicited. Symptoms of headache, visual disturbance, epigastric pain and vomiting suggest severe pre-eclampsia. On examination, oedema, particularly facial and finger oedema, would support pre-eclampsia, and hyperreflexia and ankle clonus indicate severe pre-eclampsia. Optic fundoscopy, auscultation for renal bruits (in case of renal stenosis) and palpation of the femoral pulses (to detect coarctation of the aorta) must also be performed. In addition to an MSSU and 24-hour urine collection (for creatinine clearance and protein estimation), a full blood count, clotting screen, serum urea, electrolytes, urate and liver function tests should be requested. Raised serum urate is characteristic, as is a low platelet count, abnormal clotting times and abnormal liver enzymes, in severe pre-eclampsia. The differential diagnosis includes other causes of hypertension such as renal pathology and so a renal ultrasound may be required. The fetuses may be compromised and therefore ultrasound scan examination and cardiotocography findings may alter the timing and mode of delivery. In significant pre-eclampsia, the maternal condition must be stabilised and delivery expedited. Stabilisation requires careful management of fluid balance, correction of any coagulopathy and antihypertensive treatment and anticonvulsant prophylaxis as required. In a twin pregnancy, if the first twin is cephalic and the cervix favourable, a vaginal delivery may be considered. In the absence of these favourable factors, in eclampsia or in higher-order multiple births, caesarean section is a more suitable choice. Ergometrine administration can precipitate eclampsia and should be avoided.

Comments
Pre-eclampsia is always a hot favourite of an examination question owing to its important place in the maternal mortality figures. It is therefore well worth some targeted revision.

After reading the question, underline the points that you should include in the answer, e.g. primigravida, multiple pregnancy, routine visit, 34 weeks, blood pressure of 160/100 mmHg and 2 g protein. Each of these is an important point to consider. Then concentrate on the word *justification*.

Suggested reading
Benirschke K, Kim C K 1973 Multiple pregnancy. New England Journal of Medicine 288: 1276–1284
Chamberlain G (ed) 1995 Turnbull's obstetrics. Churchill Livingstone, Edinburgh
Chamberlain G V P, Lewis P J, De Sweit M, Bulpitt C J 1978 How obstetricians manage hypertension in pregnancy. British Medical Journal 1: 626–630
Hibbard B M, Anderson M A, Drife J O et al 1996 Report on confidential enquiries into maternal deaths in the United Kingdom 1991–1993. (Triennial series) HMSO, London

4. **A primiparous woman has a stillbirth at 36 weeks' gestation. Evaluate the investigations available.**

The aim of such investigations is to determine the cause of the stillbirth, if possible, and exclude recurrent causes of stillbirth. The most important investigation is that of postmortem examination of the baby. Congenital abnormalities, such as congenital heart disease, may only be revealed during this investigation. When postmortem examination is refused by the couple, much information can still be gleaned from examination of the placenta and external examination of the fetus. The placenta may show large areas of infarction, suggestive of placental insufficiency as a cause of death. External examination may be suggestive of a particular genetic or chromosomal abnormality and X-ray examination may reveal skeletal abnormalities. Often, chromosomal analysis is not possible as the tissue samples taken (skin or cord blood) are not viable and therefore may be difficult to culture. Cord blood samples are difficult to obtain but can be tested for IgM, blood cultures, virology screen, blood typing and haemoglobin as indicated. Gestational diabetes has an association with stillbirth, but the serum blood glucose and glucose tolerance test swiftly return to normal following delivery. Fructosamine or Hb A_{1c} are of more value as they reflect the overall blood glucose control over the preceding weeks, but it is difficult to make a definitive diagnosis based on these. Kleihauer count and maternal antibody titre are important even in rhesus-positive mothers. Kleihauer count may reveal unsuspected fetomaternal haemorrhage and the antibody titre may reveal antibodies such as anti-Kell. In the absence of hydrops, it is unlikely that a virology screen such as a TORCH screen (toxoplasmosis, rubella, cytomegalovirus and herpes) would be helpful. Syphilis is now a rare disease and abnormal thyroid function is unlikely to result in stillbirth in the absence of clinical symptoms and signs, but both these conditions are important treatable causes of pregnancy loss and therefore must be considered. A screen for autoantibodies and lupus anticoagulant is of importance, particularly in cases of growth retardation.

If there are accompanying febrile symptoms, or if there is a history of ruptured membranes, an infection screen including higher vaginal, fetal and placental swabs is justified.

Comments
The question means assess the value of each investigation cited. To demonstrate that you can correctly rank the investigations in order of importance, start with the most important test – in this question the postmortem examination.

If you had difficulty with this question, revise your labour ward protocol and discuss the rationale behind each investigation with your consultant.

Suggested reading
Chamberlain G (ed) 1995 Turnbull's obstetrics. Churchill Livingstone, Edinburgh

Enkin M, Kierse M J N C 1989 Vol 1: Pregnancy. In: Chalmers I (ed) Effective care in pregnancy and childbirth. Oxford University Press, Oxford

James D K, Steer P J, Weiner C P, Gonik B (eds) 1994 High risk pregnancy – management options. Saunders, London

5. **Following two first trimester miscarriages, a 27-year-old woman presents at 8 weeks' gestation at the antenatal booking clinic. On examination, she is noted to have a goitre and exophthalmos. Explore further management.**

Maternal anxiety is likely to be high, due to the previous miscarriages. In addition to routine booking investigations and advice (such as folic acid supplementation), an ultrasound scan examination is appropriate to confirm fetal viability. This can be repeated at 12 weeks' gestation. Thyroid function tests are often unreliable in pregnancy, but in obvious clinical hyperthyroidism, thyroid function tests should be diagnostic. In equivocal tests, free T4 will confirm the diagnosis. The likely cause is Graves' disease (an autoimmune condition), but alternative diagnoses include a solitary toxic nodule, a toxic multinodular goitre or even thyrotoxicosis related to severe hyperemesis gravidarum. Clinical findings supplemented by an assay of antithyroid autoantibodies and an ultrasound scan examination of the maternal thyroid would clarify the diagnosis. Autoantibodies can cross the placenta and stimulate the fetal thyroid, resulting in fetal goitre and thyrotoxicosis. Uncontrolled maternal hyperthyroidism poses a risk to maternal health and can also result in miscarriage (a possible explanation for her two previous miscarriages). Rapid control of the thyrotoxicosis is essential and is effected by drug therapy. The antithyroid drugs propylthiouracil and carbimazole have both been used in pregnancy. As they pass the placenta, they can cause fetal goitre and hypothyroidism and so the minimum effective dosage must be used and the fetal thyroid monitored with serial ultrasound scan examination. Although abnormalities are short-lived, the thyroid function of the neonate must be monitored. As the pharmacokinetics alter throughout pregnancy and the nature of Graves' disease fluctuates, the dosage must be carefully adjusted throughout pregnancy and blocking regimes (thyroxine plus an antithyroid drug) are not used. Iodine therapy is only used preoperatively or in the advent of thyroid crisis. Propranolol is avoided because of an association with fetal growth retardation.

If medical management should fail, there is a large goitre producing pressure symptoms or there is a suspicion of malignancy, surgery may be considered. Radioactive iodine is contraindicated during pregnancy and breastfeeding as it can cause irreversible damage to the fetal thyroid.

In the event of miscarriage, investigations for recurrent miscarriage must be instigated and the thyrotoxicosis stabilised prior to further conception.

Comments
There are two issues to be explored. The first is obviously the thyrotoxicosis: the effect of pregnancy on the investigation and treatment of the thyrotoxicosis; and the effect of thyrotoxicosis and its treatment on the pregnancy. The second is the history of miscarriage. This would obviously not have been mentioned in the question unless some comment were required in the answer! However, two miscarriages was chosen so that a full discussion of recurrent miscarriage would not be indicated.

Suggested reading
James D K, Steer P J, Weiner C P, Gonik B (eds) 1994 High risk pregnancy – management options. Saunders, London
Selenkow H A 1975 Therapeutic considerations for thyrotoxicosis during pregnancy. In: Fisher D A, Burrow G N (eds) Perinatal thyroid physiology and disease. Raven Press, New York, pp 145–161
Ur E, Grossman A 1993 Thyroid disease in pregnancy. Current Obstetrics and Gynaecology 3: 145–148

PAPER 8

1. How valuable is the obstetric day care unit in current obstetric practice?

The main drive for the development of obstetric day care is to allow more women to be cared for on an outpatient basis. The major advantage is that it reduces the need for inpatient investigation and observation, thus avoiding the additional stress of the separation of the mother from the family unit. In avoiding costly inpatient stay, it can present a considerable cost saving. A wide range of women that would have been admitted to the antenatal wards may be alternatively cared for in this system. Referrals which would normally have come through the labour ward may alternatively be seen on the unit. An example would be a woman who attends with decreased fetal movements. This allows the delivery suite to concentrate on obstetric emergencies and women in labour. Obstetric day care is of particular value in the management of high-risk pregnancies as it enables those women with high-risk pregnancies to be seen outside the normal busy clinic and to have a team approach to their care. This is useful for both ensuring continuity of care and for teaching purposes.

However, in order for this system to work efficiently, the unit must be adequately staffed. A high midwife-to-patient ratio is required as the care and investigations must, of necessity, be provided in a shorter time scale. Direct access to medical staff is essential and time must be allocated within the medical staff timetable to ensure that the patients on the unit can be reviewed promptly when required. In the absence of this, the women can end up spending prolonged periods awaiting medical review. Prompt access to ultrasound scan investigation, laboratory services and cardiotocography is essential. Unless strict protocols and referral criteria are in place, the efficiency and cost-effectiveness of the unit will be affected adversely. The unit should not be used as a replacement for women who can be adequately managed in the antenatal clinic or with home visits by the community midwife.

Comments
What is the value for the woman and her family? What is the value for the staff?

Remember to consider issues such as staffing implications, cost-effectiveness, research and audit if appropriate.

Suggested reading
Draycott T J, Read M D 1996 The role of early pregnancy assessment clinics. Current Obstetrics and Gynaecology 6: 148–152
James D K, Steer P J, Weiner C P, Gonik B (eds) 1994 High risk pregnancy – management options. Saunders, London

2. An ultrasound scan examination at 24 weeks' gestation shows ascites and confirms fetal death in utero. How would you investigate the cause of this? Justify your answer.

A mid-trimester fetal loss requires careful and meticulous investigation to assess the risk to any further pregnancies, as the chance of a recurrent cause is much higher than with fetal losses in the first trimester. The presence of ascites suggests hydrops fetalis and therefore investigations relevant to this cause are important. The ultrasound scan examination may reveal fluid accumulation in other serous cavities and the fetal skin, confirming hydrops, or demonstrate a twin pregnancy, raising the possibility of a twin-to-twin transfusion. Hydrops can be categorised into immune and non-immune hydrops. Immune hydrops is classically associated with rhesus isoimmunisation (now rare). Maternal blood should be sent for blood grouping and screening for rhesus and other significant antibodies such as the anti-Kell antibodies. A Kleihauer test would indicate if there has been a fetomaternal haemorrhage, significant even in the absence of abnormal antibody levels. A direct Coombs' test and blood grouping should be performed on cord/fetal blood (post-delivery) in cases of suspected isoimmunisation.

Infection is an important cause of non-immune hydrops, justifying maternal screening for viruses such as cytomegalovirus, parvovirus B19 and rubella, as well as syphilis. Maternal diabetes and autoimmune conditions such as systemic lupus erythematosus are associated with hydrops fetalis, justifying both a diabetic (e.g. Hb A_{1c}) and an autoimmune screen. The anti-Ro antibody is particularly implicated as it causes cardiac arrhythmia. Inherited haematological conditions such as glucose-6-phosphate dehydrogenase deficiency and beta thalassaemia can cause hydrops by causing severe fetal anaemia and may be diagnosed by maternal or cord bloods.

A postmortem examination is valuable, as lethal congenital conditions causing hydrops such as cardiovascular abnormality, bladder outlet obstruction and diaphragmatic herniae are often only diagnosed in this fashion. Histological examination of the placenta may establish a placental cause for hydrops, such as chorioangioma or umbilical vein thrombosis. Karyotyping (fetal skin, blood or placenta) may reveal an associated chromosomal disorder such as Turner syndrome.

There is a strong association between non-immune hydrops fetalis and the skeletal dysplasias (although the underlying mechanism is unclear) and therefore X-ray examination of the fetus is important.

Comments

The key word is 'justify', which means that for every investigation there must be a reason or an example given.

When stuck for the causes of something, always try to organise your thoughts by using a classification, maternal/fetal etc. If you are still stuck, think back in your clinical experience. Do you remember a similar patient? How did you investigate her? Can you remember your own unit's stillbirth protocol for investigation? (You were supposed to revise it after paper 7!)

Suggested reading

Creasy R K, Resnik R (eds) 1994 Maternal–fetal medicine – principles and practice. Saunders, Philadelphia

James D K, Steer P J, Weiner C P, Gonik B (eds) 1994 High risk pregnancy – management options. Saunders, London

Johnson P, Allan L D, Maxwell D J 1993 Non immune hydrops fetalis. In: Studd J (ed) Progress in obstetrics and gynaecology. Churchill Livingstone, Edinburgh, vol 10, pp 33–50

3. **A parous woman presents at 38 weeks' gestation with a confirmed singleton breech presentation. She requests a vaginal breech delivery. How would you assess whether this mode of delivery would be feasible?**

The risk to a fetus delivering by the breech is mainly associated with asphyxia secondary to a difficult and protracted delivery. There are recognised factors associated with an increased risk of this, in particular the risk of disproportion. Assessment of the woman would be focused on these factors.

Much can be gleaned from the past obstetric history and the antenatal history of the current pregnancy. Achievement of a vaginal delivery of a term, normally grown baby would be the most important prognostic sign. The coexistence of maternal disease such as diabetes or pre-eclampsia in this pregnancy would be a relative contraindication to a vaginal delivery.

On clinical examination of the abdomen, an estimate of the fetal size and whether or not the breech was engaged would be helpful. A vaginal examination may reveal the station of the breech and what type of breech it is. An extended breech is the most favourable for a vaginal delivery. A crude clinical pelvic assessment of the pelvic diameters may be performed. An ultrasound scan reveals very important information and would confirm the clinical findings. An estimated fetal weight should be performed and the fetal attitude should be examined. It is particularly important that fetal neck extension or the presence of a footling breech should be excluded, as these are poor prognostic signs for a successful vaginal delivery.

X-ray pelvimetry is unlikely to add any information, as the past obstetric history is a more reliable indicator of pelvic size. Radiological assessment may be considered in limited circumstances, for example in a woman who has only had premature deliveries, and is better performed by computerised tomography (CT).

In the favourable circumstances described, a vaginal delivery could be considered with little excess risk to the fetus.

Continued assessment of the pregnancy is required. Engagement of the breech and the advent of normal labour is preferable to induction of labour. The continued counselling of the woman and her partner is also important, as cooperation with the advisable precautions taken with a vaginal breech delivery is also an important factor.

Comments
Remember that no points will be given for any information regarding the diagnosis, as this is already known. Therefore, answer the question with regard to assessment.

Patient choice has become an important issue in any speciality. Remember that, as an obstetrician, you have to give the best evidence and a comprehensive review. The aim is to try to help the patient to make the decision.

In your discussion, remember that the examiner may hold different views from your own, but will respect your views if supported with satisfactory evidence.

Suggested reading

Chamberlain G (ed) 1995 Turnbull's obstetrics. Churchill Livingstone, Edinburgh

Enkin M, Kierse M J N C 1989 Vol 1: Pregnancy. In: Chalmers I (ed) Effective care in pregnancy and childbirth. Oxford University Press, Oxford

James D K, Steer P J, Weiner C P, Gonik B (eds) 1994 High risk pregnancy – management options. Saunders, London

4. **A 35-year-old woman presents at 30 weeks' gestation in her second pregnancy for a routine antenatal visit. It is noted that 3 years previously she had a subarachnoid haemorrhage. Debate your management.**

It would be essential to ascertain the cause of the subarachnoid haemorrhage. Details from the previous medical records, from the patient and from her previous medical team must be obtained and the opinion of the neurosurgical team sought. The main concern would be that of a further subarachnoid haemorrhage and advice would be sought as to what risk labour would pose.

A history of a traumatic subarachnoid would indicate a very low risk of further problems. If the aetiology was that of a ruptured berry aneurysm, then the major risk does occur in later pregnancy, but rupture is unusual during labour. If the aneurysm has been operated on surgically, this would still further decrease the risk, and as the incident was 3 years ago, this would also indicate a low risk. The existence of multiple aneurysms would, however, be a cause for concern. An arteriovenous malformation conversely has a high chance of rupture in labour and the puerperium and if it has not been operated on, poses a significant risk. Some authorities have even advocated neurosurgical correction electively during pregnancy.

In the case of an uncorrected arteriovenous malformation, a labour with good analgesia and an assisted delivery or a caesarean section should be performed. This should also be considered in cases of multiple berry aneurysms. The existence of coexisting obstetric problems would lower the threshold for caesarean section still further.

Particular care should be taken to assess any residual neurological deficit and disability which have implications for her care during labour and delivery. If there is significant disability, care must be taken to ensure that the correct support network is available on discharge to provide care for mother and child. This will involve communication with both the primary care team and paediatric colleagues.

Comments

Remember, as with all medical problems, to discuss the effect of the condition on the pregnancy and vice versa. The implications for delivery, anaesthesia, etc. are important here.

The question omits whether or not this woman has any residual

problems. In any case in which the woman is disabled, it is impoi
mention the extra support the family may need.

Suggested reading

Chamberlain G (ed) 1995 Turnbull's obstetrics. Churchill Livingstone,
   Edinburgh
Enkin M, Kierse M J N C 1989 Vol 1: Pregnancy. In: Chalmers I (ed)
   Effective care in pregnancy and childbirth. Oxford University Press,
   Oxford
James D K, Steer P J, Weiner C P, Gonik B (eds) 1994 High risk
   pregnancy – management options. Saunders, London

5. **A 30-year-old parous woman is referred by her general practitioner
   at 27 weeks' gestation with jaundice. Account for your strategy to
   reach a diagnosis.**

The jaundice may be secondary to the pregnancy or incidental to the
pregnancy. A full history should be taken and a full clinical examination
performed. The history should include enquiry regarding the incidence
of headache, abdominal pain, visual disturbance and vomiting. Foreign
travel, sexual contacts and contact with infectious jaundice, alcohol
consumption, substance abuse and previous blood transfusion must be
enquired about. A family history of jaundice may also be relevant.
Jaundice can be secondary to therapeutic interventions such as
medication or anaesthetics (such as halothane). The examination
would include the signs of pre-eclampsia (oedema, hypertension,
epigastric tenderness, hyperreflexia), but careful palpation for a liver
edge would be performed. The presence of Murphy's sign suggests
cholecystitis. If appropriate, signs of liver failure should be elicited,
such as hepatic flap. Palmar erythema and spider naevi are present in
normal pregnancy and are therefore unhelpful. The urine should be
tested for bilirubin and urobilinogen. Investigations would include a full
blood count, urea and electrolytes, liver function tests, viral screen for
hepatitis A, B and C (others if indicated) and a clotting profile. A
macrocytic anaemia may indicate alcohol consumption. Conjugated
bilirubin suggests an extrahepatic cause. Subsequently an ultrasound
of the liver, gall bladder and biliary tree is essential. This would
demonstrate the presence of gallstones and examination of the liver
would demonstrate any parenchymal disease, such as cirrhosis or
intrahepatic tumours. Other modalities of imaging are relatively
contraindicated except that of magnetic resonance imaging (MRI). The
indications are that MRI, whilst being apparently safe in pregnancy,
allows superior imaging. Liver biopsy can be performed in the absence
of a clotting abnormality, but is rarely required. Although conditions
such as intrahepatic cholestasis, pre-eclampsia and acute fatty liver
could occur at this gestation, typically they occur later in the third
trimester. At this gestation, infectious hepatitis and gallstones are the
most likely diagnoses.

Comments

The question does not specify investigations, therefore it is important to
discuss the importance of history and examination findings.

Classify causes into non-obstetric and obstetric. Remember to emphasise the importance of multidisciplinary input.

Suggested reading
Chamberlain G (ed) 1995 Turnbull's obstetrics. Churchill Livingstone, Edinburgh
James D K, Steer P J, Weiner C P, Gonik B (eds) 1994 High risk pregnancy – management options. Saunders, London
Nelson-Piercy C 1997 Liver disease in pregnancy. Current Obstetrics and Gynaecology 7: 36–42

PAPER 9

1. **An obese 35-year-old primigravida is found to have two episodes of glycosuria in the second trimester. Justify your approach to the management of the remainder of her pregnancy.**

This woman has significant diabetic risk factors, in view of the obesity, maternal age and two episodes of glycosuria. The family history (diabetes, high-birth-weight babies) may lend further weight to this. Undetected gestational diabetes is associated with poor outcome and therefore screening is essential by random or fasting blood glucose, blood glucose profile or glucose tolerance test. In this woman with significant risk factors, a glucose tolerance test using a 75-g oral load is appropriate. If this is normal, the cause may be renal glycosuria, but if glycosuria persists it would be prudent to repeat the glucose tolerance test. Similarly a borderline result should be repeated later in pregnancy, but such a result, in conjunction with the woman's obesity, would support referral to the dietitian.

Glucose measurement of greater than 11 mmol/L 2 hours post-challenge would indicate frank gestational diabetes, whereas 8–11 mmol/L supports the diagnosis of impaired glucose tolerance. These cases should be managed in conjunction with the diabetologists, specialist nurse and paediatricians. In impaired glucose tolerance and diabetes, a low-sugar diet and blood glucose monitoring are mandatory. Insulin is occasionally used in impaired glucose tolerance (dependent on the blood glucose profile), but it is the treatment of first choice in gestational diabetes as it allows tight control of blood glucose levels and oral hypoglycaemics are known to cross the placenta. Clinical examination and serial ultrasound scan examinations may detect polyhydramnios and macrosomia characteristic of poor diabetic control. Interpretation of biophysical scoring must take into account that an increase in liquor volume improving the score is actually associated with increased risk. A Doppler scan examination is also of limited benefit. Preterm delivery is often necessary in cases of poor diabetic control. In the absence of complications, the aim would still be to deliver those women with glucose intolerance or diabetes prior to the expected date of delivery. In the case of a markedly macrosomic child, delivery by caesarean section should be considered.

Comments

The mention of the multidisciplinary approach to the management of this relatively common condition is a must in any general medical condition, to demonstrate that you are in tune with current thinking. Other examples would be epilepsy, thyrotoxicosis, prolactinoma, etc.

Note that the wording of the question confines the answer to the pregnancy. Postpartum follow-up and future pregnancy are excluded.

Suggested reading

Chamberlain G (ed) 1995 Turnbull's obstetrics. Churchill Livingstone, Edinburgh
James D K, Steer P J, Weiner C P, Gonik B (eds) 1994 High risk pregnancy – management options. Saunders, London

Vaughan N J A 1994 Diabetes in pregnancy. Current Obstetrics and
Gynaecology 4: 155–159

2. Critically review the role of ultrasound scan examination in modern obstetrics.

Although ultrasound scan examination has been considered to be a huge asset in obstetrics, there has been concern regarding its possible misuse, resulting in anxiety and undue exposure of the fetus.

In the first trimester, ultrasound (particularly transvaginal) has been invaluable in establishing viability and location of pregnancy and the diagnosis of trophoblastic disease. In the second trimester, the main use is for anomaly screening. The initial excitement regarding the discovery of markers for chromosomal disorders has been tempered by the knowledge that these soft markers can cause undue maternal stress unless accompanied by adequate counselling. Ultrasound reduces the chance of undiagnosed multiple pregnancy and allows chorionicity to be determined. Ultrasound has enabled rapid progress in invasive procedures such as amniocentesis, chorionic villous sampling and cordocentesis. In the second trimester, however, Doppler ultrasound auscultation can confirm viability. In the third trimester, ultrasound scan examination can locate placental site and be used to monitor high-risk pregnancy (intrauterine growth retardation, diabetic pregnancy and multiple pregnancy).

Serial biometry and the biophysical profile have become important tools in modern obstetrics, scan estimation of liquor volume being a particularly important prognostic indicator. However, Doppler ultrasound (with the exception of absent or reduced end-diastolic flow) does not appear to be of additional value in clinical management of high-risk pregnancy. Definitive antenatal confirmation of intrauterine fetal death has been possible with the advent of ultrasound, allowing better preparation, counselling and appropriate management.

Intrapartum ultrasound can be used to demonstrate fetal presentation. In antepartum haemorrhage, the placental site can be confirmed, but placental abruption is rarely seen on ultrasound scan. On labour wards, the presence of a portable ultrasound machine has facilitated rapid decisions. However, adequate training is paramount as misdiagnosis in this setting can have grave consequences.

Throughout pregnancy, ultrasound may be crucial in the diagnosis of coexistent pathology such as ovarian cysts or uterine fibroids. Doppler ultrasound may be safely used to investigate deep vein thrombosis. In the puerperium, retained products of conception may be demonstrated on ultrasound scan examination, though in the first 2 weeks it is not a specific test.

Comments

Ultrasound scan examination has a changing role throughout pregnancy, therefore it is best to approach the question by analysing its role in the first, second, third trimester, intrapartum and postpartum. Note that the question is not confined to antenatal ultrasound scan.

Don't forget to include the role of different types of ultrasound scan examination: Doppler, transvaginal, etc.

Suggested reading

Bakketeig L S, Erik-Nes S H, Jacobson G et al 1984 Randomised controlled trial of ultrasonographic screening in pregnancy. Lancet 2: 207–211

Bennet M J, Little G, Dewhurst J et al 1982 Predictive value of ultrasound measurement in early pregnancy: a randomised controlled trial. British Journal of Obstetrics and Gynaecology 89: 338–341

Chamberlain G (ed) 1995 Turnbull's obstetrics. Churchill Livingstone, Edinburgh

3. **An unbooked 26-year-old woman presents in advanced labour at term. She admits to a history of drug addiction. How would you conduct her care?**

An unbooked woman presenting in labour is a far from ideal situation. *Development of rapport* with a woman established in labour, who has not had any antenatal preparation, can be difficult. There are several additional considerations in this case. Good communication between the medical staff and patient is essential, to get as accurate a picture as possible regarding the type, quantity and method of administration of her drug addiction. A plan can then be formulated so that the risk of drug withdrawal can be minimised. Acute withdrawal state can not only lead to difficulties with management of the woman, but can be life-threatening to the fetus. In opiate abuse, adequate replacement must be given. Pethidine or diamorphine may be used for analgesia and will also provide replacement, but they are unlikely to be adequate for analgesia, and epidural anaesthesia may be required. Following a full history and examination, specific investigations may be indicated. As a minimum, routine antenatal booking investigations should be completed. In particular, blood group and a full blood count should be obtained urgently. Hepatitis B and human immunodeficiency virus (HIV) screening would not be performed at this time, as adequate counselling is not possible in this situation, but may be considered postnatally. In the case of intravenous drug abusers, it is advisable to obtain venous access in case of difficulties procuring access in an emergency. If available, a portable scan may add to the assessment of the fetal condition and presentation and exclude multiple pregnancy. Continuous cardiotocographic monitoring should be instituted, as the risk of fetal distress is higher in this group. The paediatricians should be informed from the outset, so there is time to counsel the mother regarding the likely fetal outcome and to allow preparations for delivery. No Narcan must be given to the baby at birth, owing to the risk of abrupt opiate withdrawal, which can lead to neonatal death. As the woman's hepatitis B and HIV status are unknown, there should be careful adherence to local protocols to reduce the risk of patient-to-staff transmission.

Comments

Your answer must be mainly concerned with the specific problems associated with drug addiction. This involves your approach to tackling the problems associated with the intrapartum care of the woman, the implications for the neonate and the implications for the staff.

There will also be marks allocated for details regarding the problems posed by any unbooked woman presenting in advanced labour.

Remember the 'safe doctor' point of not giving naloxone to the neonate if the woman is addicted to opiates.

Suggested reading
Beeley L, Stirrat G M (eds) 1986 Prescribing in pregnancy. In: Clinics in obstetrics and gynaecology. Saunders, Eastbourne

Chamberlain G (ed) 1995 Turnbull's obstetrics. Churchill Livingstone, Edinburgh

James D K, Steer P J, Weiner C P, Gonik B (eds) 1994 High risk pregnancy – management options. Saunders, London

4. **Review the principles and recent developments regarding rhesus prophylaxis.**

The aim of rhesus prophylaxis is to reduce the risk of a woman who has a rhesus-negative blood group developing antibodies to her rhesus-positive child, resulting in rhesus disease. The blood groups associated with this are D, c and e. The main offender is D as it is the most immunogenic. If a few fetal red blood cells of a group D (rhesus-positive) baby pass through the placenta into the maternal (group d) circulation, this stimulates the maternal immune system to produce anti-D antibodies. These antibodies can pass the placenta and in sufficient quantities (not usually in the first pregnancy) may result in significant haemolysis of fetal red blood cells, leading to anaemia and neonatal jaundice or even hydrops fetalis and intrauterine death. To prevent the sensitisation of rhesus-negative women during pregnancy, the fetus is assumed to be rhesus positive. Anti-D is given after any situation in which fetomaternal haemorrhage may have occurred, e.g. antepartum haemorrhage or amniocentesis. At delivery, the baby's blood group is checked by cord bloods and anti-D (250 iu prior to 20 weeks' gestation, 500 iu after) is given if the baby is rhesus positive. The administered anti-D destroys the fetal red blood cells before the maternal immune system is triggered. A Kleihauer test gives some indication of the size of a fetomaternal haemorrhage, allowing further anti-D to be given if indicated. Since the introduction of this policy, the incidence of rhesus sensitisation has plummeted and with it the associated perinatal mortality. However, there are still some women who become sensitised, despite careful adherence to this protocol, due to silent transplacental haemorrhage. Recent trials using further doses of anti-D antenatally, at 28 and 34 weeks for example, have suggested that this would allow still further reduction and this concept was endorsed by the 1997 RCOG/RCP Consensus Conference in Edinburgh. The potential problems of cost-effectiveness, the risk of transmission of viral infections (as anti-D is a blood product) and procurement of supplies will need to be fully addressed before this is adopted into the current protocol.

Comments
The first part of the question is a straightforward, factual account of the current practice in rhesus prophylaxis. However, the second part requires a critical appraisal of the proposals for routine antenatal prophylaxis.

Use of a blood product always raises concerns regarding safety (viral agents) and cost-effectiveness.

Suggested reading

Bowman J M 1984 Rhesus haemolytic disease. In: Wald N J (ed) Antenatal and neonatal screening. Oxford University Press, Oxford, pp 314–344

Chamberlain G (ed) 1995 Turnbull's obstetrics. Churchill Livingstone, Edinburgh

James D K, Steer P J, Weiner C P, Gonik B (eds) 1994 High risk pregnancy – management options. Saunders, London

Royal College of Physicians of Edinburgh/Royal College of Obstetricians and Gynaecologists 1997 Consensus Conference on anti-D prophylaxis. Journal of Obstetrics and Gynaecology 17(4): 420–421

5. **Compare and contrast the anticonvulsant agents available for the prevention of eclamptic fits.**

Many drugs have been used and still are used in an attempt to prevent eclamptic fits. The reason for this plurality is because no one agent has been shown to have been fully effective, nor is any one agent free of side-effects.

The traditional agents, intravenous diazepam and chlormethiazole edisylate, have waned in popularity. Both are very effective in initial rapid control in cases of imminent eclampsia, but they are less effective than other agents in long-term usage. Both are associated with apnoea and hypotension and therefore require close monitoring. They should not be used where mechanical ventilation is not available. Chlormethiazole has, however, a short half-life and therefore can be carefully titrated against the patient's requirements. The fear of benzodiazepine overdose has lessened since the introduction of the selective reversal reagent, flumazenil. Paraldehyde is now only used intramuscularly. It is rarely used, but it may have a role during transfers from areas remote from hospital care. The commonest agent in this country is phenytoin. Although more effective than the previously mentioned agents, it requires some time to administer, making it unsuitable for emergency control. The dosage has to be carefully calculated according to body weight and given under careful supervision and cardiac monitoring. It is, however, quite well established in use in Britain in obstetrics, which enhances its safety. Magnesium sulphate, however, has not as yet gained in popularity to the same degree. Widely used in the USA, it has been shown to be effective in the prevention of eclampsia and is thought to pass the blood–brain barrier to a greater extent than phenytoin. It is administered under close supervision under cardiac monitoring and careful observation of deep tendon reflexes. Loss of deep tendon reflexes heralds toxicity, which can be associated with an altered conscious state and even coma. Toxicity effects can be reversed with calcium gluconate, unlike phenytoin.

Comments

The question means discuss the similarities (compare) and the differences (contrast) in the characteristics of the commonly used agents.

Write an equivalent essay plan for the antihypertensive agents commonly used in pre-eclampsia.

Suggested reading

Dommisse J 1990 Phenytoin sodium and magnesium sulphate in the management of eclampsia. British Journal of Obstetrics and Gynaecology 97: 104–109

Duley L 1996 Magnesium sulphate regimens for women with eclampsia: message from the Collaborative Eclampsia Trial. British Journal of Obstetrics and Gynaecology 103: 103–105

James D K, Steer P J, Weiner C P, Gonik B (eds) 1994 High risk pregnancy – management options. Saunders, London

Mackenzie F, Greer I A 1996 Preventing eclampsia. Current Obstetrics and Gynaecology 6: 159–164

Rosevear S K, Stirrat G M 1996 Handbook of obstetric management. Blackwell Science, Oxford

PAPER 10

1. **At 30 weeks' gestation, an ultrasound scan examination reveals a major degree of placenta praevia. Justify your management plan for the remainder of the pregnancy.**

An increasing number of women are being diagnosed as having placenta praevia whilst asymptomatic, due to the increasing use of ultrasound scan examinations. Full comprehension of the problem by the patient is difficult to achieve when there have been no episodes of antepartum haemorrhage (one-third of cases). Careful counselling is mandatory in all cases of placenta praevia, but particularly in this subset of patients, to ensure compliance to the management plan. An episode of bleeding, particularly if in the second trimester, is associated with a worse outcome. Traditional management would involve admission for bed rest in the third trimester and would be appropriate in patients who have experienced an antepartum haemorrhage. In asymptomatic women, the impact on the family must be weighed against the woman's capacity to receive rapid obstetric care in case of haemorrhage. The presence of concurrent obstetric complications such as twin pregnancy and diabetes (both associated with placenta praevia) would decrease the threshold for admission.

Antenatal steroids should be given, as the chance of rapid premature delivery is high. These neonates are considered to be at increased risk of RDS, owing to the absence of intrauterine stress to mature the lungs.

Care must be taken to maintain the woman's haemoglobin, to increase her ability to withstand a bleed. Iron deficiency should be corrected and transfusion performed if required. Cross-matched blood should be available at all times, in case of haemorrhage.

Serial scanning to localise the placenta is justified, as growth of the lower segment in the third trimester can lead to apparent migration of the placenta. This does not occur significantly past 38 weeks and therefore a decision can be made in the asymptomatic patient at this time. With the advent of high-resolution scanning, there is no place for examination in theatre to localise the placenta: a hazardous procedure which converts an elective procedure to an emergency delivery.

In the event of continuous or heavy bleeding, expectant management would be abandoned and delivery sought. Delivery would also be expedited in cases of premature labour. Beta adrenoceptor agonists would be contraindicated as they reduce the ability of the woman to compensate for haemorrhage. In a major degree of placenta praevia, delivery must be by caesarean section. Attempted vaginal delivery would be associated with heavy vaginal bleeding. Caesarean section should be performed by a senior obstetrician. An anterior placenta praevia can cause technical difficulties in accessing the uterus and increased haemorrhage. This, coupled with an area of accretia classically associated with a previous caesarean section scar, is extremely hazardous and has a high caesarean hysterectomy rate: 16% in one series. A classical caesarean section may be required in premature delivery. A general anaesthetic is preferable, due to the increased operative difficulty. Postpartum haemorrhage is common, due to the decreased ability of the lower segment to contract and staunch the bleeding from the placental bed. A high dose of oxytocic infusion is required.

Comments
Discussion points include inpatient versus outpatient management and the role of ultrasound scan, examination in theatre, etc.

Remember to emphasise the safety aspects, cross-matching of blood, operation by an experienced surgeon and, importantly, no vaginal examinations!

Suggested reading
Chamberlain G (ed) 1995 Turnbull's obstetrics. Churchill Livingstone, Edinburgh

Hibbard B M, Anderson M A, Drife J O et al 1996 Report on confidential enquiries into maternal deaths in the United Kingdom 1991–1993. (Triennial series) HMSO, London

James D K, Steer P J, Weiner C P, Gonik B (eds) 1994 High risk pregnancy – management options. Saunders, London

Rosevear S K, Stirrat G M 1996 Handbook of obstetric management. Blackwell Science, Oxford

2. What information do you gain from macroscopic examination of a placenta?

Examination of the placenta is a mandatory part of the management of any delivery, as the information gleaned from the placenta is extensive. On the labour ward, a careful macroscopic examination would begin with the weighing of the placenta. Taking gestational age into account, a small placenta is suggestive of intrauterine growth retardation, whereas a larger placenta may be seen in diabetic pregnancies. Although not completely reliable, examination can reveal whether the placenta appears complete or incomplete. Obviously, the concern if the placenta appears incomplete is that fragments of the placenta are retained in the uterus. The morphological appearance of the placenta can be of no clinical significance (battledore placenta) or be highly significant, such as placenta succenturiata. The latter is associated with a high incidence of a retained lobe of placenta. Examination of the placenta may reveal vessels running in the membranes, for example in a placenta velamentosa. These may form vasa praevia and may provide an explanation for a baby born in an unexpectedly poor condition. Pallor of the placenta may suggest fetomaternal haemorrhage. A retroplacental clot would confirm a placental abruption. Placental infarctions are of significance when covering a large proportion of the placenta as they interfere with placental function and therefore are associated with intrauterine growth retardation. A hydropic appearance would be suggestive of hydrops fetalis. Placental tumours can also be found, although rare. The presence of odour and exudate of the placental membranes are found in cases of chorioamnionitis. Examination of the cord is important. A true knot in the cord may provide some explanation for fetal distress, whereas the presence of a single umbilical artery is associated with a higher incidence of congenital abnormality. Examination of the placenta is essential in multiple pregnancy, as determination of the chorionicity can confirm that the babies are identical. Injection of dye into placental vasculature of one twin can demonstrate the presence of anastomosis leading to twin-to-twin transfusion. It has been suggested that examination of the placenta may even predict health in later life.

Comments
This type of question tests core obstetrics knowledge, therefore the standard expected will be high. A systematic approach to ensure a comprehensive answer is essential.

There is no excuse for forgetting the basics. If you forget to mention checking that the placenta is complete, you are likely to be penalised.

Suggested reading
Chamberlain G (ed) 1995 Turnbull's obstetrics. Churchill Livingstone, Edinburgh

Dearden L, Ockleford C D 1983 Structure of human trophoblast: correlation with function. In: Loke C, White H (eds) Biology of trophoblast. Elsevier, London, pp 69–110

Fox H 1998 Abnormal placentation. Current Obstetrics and Gynaecology 8: 21–26

3. **At 34 weeks' gestation, a primigravida presents with a generalised seizure. Outline your proposed management.**

Initial management must concentrate on stabilisation of the woman. If the woman is still fitting at the time of presentation, the airway must be secured and inhalation prevented by positioning the woman on her side, head down and utilising oropharyngeal suction. Oxygen therapy should be given and intravenous access secured. An intravenous bolus of diazepam is the drug of first choice to stop generalised fit. If there is no response, the anaesthetist should be called, as barbiturate anaesthesia is indicated whatever the underlying pathology. Monitoring by pulse oximetry, electrocardiograph, automated blood pressure recording and a cardiotocograph is appropriate. Assessment of the woman should follow, to determine the cause of the fit. The history may have to be gleaned from relatives and the medical notes. There may be a history of epilepsy and she may already be on prophylactic medication. A past history of drug or alcohol abuse, or symptoms suggestive of intracranial pathology such as a cerebrovascular accident may be significant. Multidisciplinary input would be appropriate in these cases. In the absence of such a history, the most likely cause would be eclampsia. Examination findings of oedema, hypertension and proteinuria (by a catheter specimen) would support the diagnosis. A longer-acting agent should be given to prevent further fits. Magnesium sulphate is the agent of choice, but where this is unavailable, phenytoin can be selected. Emergency control of the blood pressure can be achieved by a slow intravenous bolus of hydralazine, followed by a maintenance infusion of hydralazine or labetalol. A urinary catheter and central venous line are inserted to allow strict monitoring of fluid balance. In significant oliguria or anuria, an infusion of albumin may be used in accordance with the central venous pressure. In cases of eclampsia, prompt delivery must be accomplished. If the woman is stable and the cervix favourable, induction of labour may be contemplated. In a primigravid woman at 34 weeks' gestation, it is likely that the delivery would be by caesarean section. Ergometrine-containing drugs would be avoided as they can precipitate further eclampsia. Close monitoring is essential in the early puerperium.

Comments
Remember emergency management first.

Classify the causes into obstetric and non-obstetric and discuss the importance of multidisciplinary input.

Suggested reading
Chamberlain G (ed) 1995 Turnbull's obstetrics. Churchill Livingstone, Edinburgh

Hibbard B M, Anderson M A, Drife J O et al 1996 Report on confidential enquiries into maternal deaths in the United Kingdom 1991–1993. (Triennial series) HMSO, London

James D K, Steer P J, Weiner C P, Gonik B (eds) 1994 High risk pregnancy – management options. Saunders, London

Rosevear S K, Stirrat G M 1996 Handbook of obstetric management. Blackwell Science, Oxford

4. **A 35-year-old presents with excessive vomiting and 8 weeks' amenorrhoea. Discuss your management.**

The most likely diagnosis would be hyperemesis gravidarum. A full history should be taken, concentrating on the possibility of pregnancy, including vaginal bleeding, urinary symptoms and gastrointestinal symptoms, as a urinary tract infection and gastroenteritis are the common differential diagnoses. Drug ingestion is also associated with hyperemesis gravidarum. Of particular importance is the amount and nature of oral intake: this, accompanied by clinical examination, can be used to assess the degree of nutrition and dehydration. A pregnancy test, pelvic examination or ultrasound scan examination will confirm the diagnosis of pregnancy.

The urine should be checked for ketones (an indication of dehydration) and protein, suggestive of a urinary tract infection (UTI). A midstream specimen of urine should be sent for culture. Blood should be taken for urea and electrolytes. A raised urea would be indicative of dehydration. In prolonged vomiting, thyroid function and liver function can be deranged and must be checked. A full blood count may reveal a raised white cell count, suggestive of infection such as a UTI.

An ultrasound scan examination may reveal a multiple pregnancy or hydatidiform mole, both associated with hyperemesis gravidarum, because of the high circulating values of human chorionic gonadotrophin.

In cases where oral uptake is compromised, admission for rehydration is advised. An intravenous infusion (IVI) would be sited and the patient's oral intake restricted to sips of fluid until the nausea had settled. The well-established anti-emetics (e.g. metoclopramide) may be used.

Conservative management is all that is usually required. Advice to take regular carbohydrate snacks rather than full meals may allow women to cope at home. By 12 weeks, the majority of cases will have settled. In those cases which have not settled, a trial of other agents such as intravenous steroids has been used. Prolonged vomiting can lead to depletion of vitamin levels. This leads to an increased risk of folic acid deficiency and therefore neural tube defects. Cases of Wernicke's encephalopathy have also been described. Parenteral vitamins should be considered in these cases. In some extreme cases, termination of pregnancy has been performed.

Comments
Note that the question does not say hyperemesis gravidarum and therefore you must include a differential diagnosis and appropriate investigations.
  Don't forget to discuss the long-term concerns if this problem does not settle. The question is not restricted to management of the acute episode.

Suggested reading
Chamberlain G (ed) 1995 Turnbull's obstetrics. Churchill Livingstone, Edinburgh
James D K, Steer P J, Weiner C P, Gonik B (eds) 1994 High risk pregnancy – management options. Saunders, London
Rosevear S K, Stirrat G M 1996 Handbook of obstetric management. Blackwell Science, Oxford
Nelson-Piercy C 1997 Hyperemesis gravidarum. Current Obstetrics and Gynaecology 7: 98–103

5. **Following an uneventful antenatal course, a routine full blood count at 28 weeks' gestation reveals a platelet count of 56 × 10⁹/L. Formulate a management plan for the remainder of the pregnancy.**

Antenatal management would initially focus on the establishment of a diagnosis. The differential diagnosis to be considered would depend on whether there were other significant features or this was an isolated finding. In this case, the platelet count seems to be an isolated finding and the individual asymptomatic, but underlying pathology such as pre-eclamptic toxaemia, systemic lupus erythematosus, non-specific marrow suppression due to infection and neoplastic marrow infiltration must still be considered. The blood count may reveal a profound megaloblastic anaemia. Treatment of this, for example with folic acid, will cause rapid reversal. The two most likely primary conditions in such a case are benign gestational thrombocytopenia and maternal immune thrombocytopenia. Multidisciplinary input from haematologists, paediatricians and anaesthetists is important. The platelet count must be monitored with serial full blood counts. As the pregnancy was 'uneventful', it is likely that the booking platelet count was normal. This would suggest benign gestational thrombocytopenia, although it would be unusual for the platelets to drop to this level. Gestational thrombocytopenia and autoimmune thrombocytopenia can be differentiated by autoantibody screening. Antenatally, management would depend on the problems experienced. Platelet infusion would be considered in the case of spontaneous bruising and bleeding or a platelet count below $50 \times 10^9/L$ near term. In autoimmune thrombocytopenia, platelet infusion can exacerbate the problem by exciting an increased platelet response, so antenatal steroids and intravenous immunoglobulin are preferred. In autoimmune thrombocytopenia, the autoantibodies can be IgG, pass the placenta and put the neonate at risk of intracranial bleeding. Procedures such as ventouse and fetal blood sampling must be avoided and cord bloods taken to screen the baby.

In all cases of thrombocytopenia, epidural anaesthesia and spinal anaesthesia should be avoided, in view of the risk of haematoma formation. An uncomplicated vaginal delivery is the safest form of delivery for both mother and baby. Delivery by caesarean section should be reserved for obstetric indications. Cross-matched blood and platelets should be available. Owing to the increased risk of haemorrhage, soft tissue damage should be avoided, prompt perineal repair effected and the third stage actively managed.

Comments

The management is obviously dependent on the aetiology. Your answer would sensibly start with this, followed by a discussion of risk reduction for mother and for the fetus.

Be careful to emphasise the potential risk associated with regional anaesthesia and operative delivery for the mother and particularly the ventouse and fetal blood sampling for the fetus.

Suggested reading

Chamberlain G (ed) 1995 Turnbull's obstetrics. Churchill Livingstone, Edinburgh

James D K, Steer P J, Weiner C P, Gonik B (eds) 1994 High risk pregnancy – management options. Saunders, London

Letsky E A, Greaves M 1996 Guidelines on the investigation and management of thrombocytopenia in pregnancy and neonatal alloimmune thrombocytopenia. British Journal of Haematology 95: 21–26

GYNAECOLOGY

Gynaecology Questions

1. A 32-year-old nulliparous woman has long-standing confirmed polycystic ovarian syndrome (PCOS). When attending clinic she states that she intends to stop the combined oral contraceptive pill to conceive. How would you proceed with her care?

2. Evaluate the range of surgical options available for the treatment of genuine stress incontinence (GSI). On what criteria would you base your selection of an appropriate operation?

3. All menopausal women should be on hormone replacement therapy (HRT). Critically appraise this statement.

4. A 40-year-old woman is referred by her general practitioner with a single mildly dyskaryotic cervical smear. Critically appraise the options for her care.

5. At 9 weeks and after slight vaginal bleeding, an ultrasound scan confirms the presence of a missed abortion. Compare and contrast possible courses of action.

PAPER 2

1. Review the recent advances and probable future developments in contraception.

2. A 24-year-old woman has persistent vaginal bleeding following a dilatation and curettage for gestational trophoblastic tumour (GTT). Give a detailed account of your management.

3. Following a total abdominal hysterectomy and bilateral salpingo-oophorectomy for endometriosis, a 39-year-old woman presents with continuous urinary incontinence. How would you assess this problem?

4. A 35-year-old woman presents with amenorrhoea and vasomotor symptoms. Subsequent serum follicle stimulating hormone (FSH) and luteinising hormone (LH) levels are markedly raised. Explore further management.

5. How would you construct and implement a unit policy for thromboembolic prophylaxis for gynaecological surgery?

PAPER 3

1. Critically evaluate the current controversies in the field of assisted reproduction.

2. A 19-year-old woman presents with lower abdominal pain associated with vaginal discharge, both of 8 days' duration. Because of worsening pain and a pyrexia, her general practitioner has sought a gynaecological opinion. How would you proceed with her care?

3. A 17-year-old girl presents with primary amenorrhoea. How would you reach a diagnosis?

4. Evaluate the place of laparoscopy in current gynaecological practice.

5. A 47-year-old woman has a hysterectomy due to intractable menorrhagia. The subsequent histology report reads as follows: 'Uterus: within the cavity of the uterus is a well differentiated adenocarcinoma. This tumour infiltrates the myometrium, but this is superficial, being confined to the inner one-third of the myometrium'. How would you conduct her subsequent care?

PAPER 4

1. All gynaecological malignancies should be treated in specialised centres. Critically appraise this statement.

2. An 11-year-old girl presents with vaginal bleeding following a fall. How would you approach her care?

3. A 50-year-old lady presents with a 2-year history of worsening stress and urge incontinence. Consider the options for further investigation of this problem.

4. A 32-year-old woman presents with primary infertility. A laparoscopic survey reveals endometriosis. Critically evaluate the management options.

5. A primiparous woman presents 2 months postnatally, complaining of persistent dyspareunia. Explore further management.

PAPER 5

1. How can we avoid litigation in gynaecological surgery?
2. Critically appraise the treatment options for a confirmed tubal pregnancy.
3. What impact has the advent of evidence-based practice had on the management of menorrhagia?
4. A 36-year-old woman has dysfunctional uterine bleeding. She expresses a wish to avoid hysterectomy. Evaluate the range of treatment options available.
5. An obese 34-year-old woman was referred by her general practitioner because of oligomenorrhoea and excessive hair growth. Outline further management.

PAPER 6

1. A 5-year-old girl presents with a 2-week history of offensive profuse vaginal discharge. Justify your management strategy.

2. Evaluate the place of the menorrhagia clinic in modern gynaecological practice.

3. During ovulation induction, a 34-year-old woman becomes ill and collapses. How would you approach subsequent management?

4. A 25-year-old woman presents requesting sterilisation. Discuss her preoperative management and counselling.

5. A 60-year-old widow presents with recurrent offensive vaginal discharge. Discuss the further management of this case.

PAPER 7

1. Debate the impact of the early pregnancy assessment unit.

2. A 74-year-old woman has confirmed advanced ovarian carcinoma. How would you approach her care?

3. A 17-year-old girl presents 14 hours after unprotected intercourse, requesting help. How would you proceed to manage this problem?

4. Review the treatment options available for premenstrual syndrome.

5. Following a total abdominal hysterectomy and bilateral salpingo-oophorectomy, a 49-year-old woman presents with vaginal vault prolapse. Explore further management.

PAPER 8

1. A 38-year-old woman presents, worried about the chances of developing ovarian carcinoma. Her mother, and more recently her sister, have died of ovarian carcinoma in their 40s. How would you counsel her?

2. A 19-year-old woman presents requesting oral contraception. She has insulin-dependent diabetes mellitus, but is well controlled. Can you justify giving it to her?

3. Evaluate the role of vaginal hysterectomy in modern gynaecological practice.

4. A 30-year-old woman has persistent pelvic pain and dyspareunia. A diagnostic laparoscopy reveals extensive active endometriosis, including involvement of the left ovary. Evaluate the treatment options.

5. A girl of 7 years presents with full development of secondary female sexual characteristics. Discuss further management.

PAPER 9

1. A 59-year-old woman was referred by her general practitioner, who noticed a marked cystourethrocoele when taking a routine cervical smear. Justify your further management.

2. A 40-year-old woman is found to have stage 1b carcinoma of the cervix. Describe how this staging would have been reached and critically discuss the options for management.

3. Critically evaluate the role of a routine 6 week postoperative hospital visit following major gynaecological surgery.

4. A 28-year-old woman presents with her husband of 1 year's standing, having been unable to consummate their marriage. How would you manage this problem?

5. During routine investigations for infertility, a hysterosalpingogram shows a hypoplastic uterus and absent right tube. Explore the management options.

PAPER 10

1. Minimal-access surgery should replace open surgery in gynaecological practice. Critically evaluate this statement.

2. A 20-year-old mentally retarded woman attends the clinic requesting contraceptive advice. Compare management strategies.

3. A 44-year-old woman presents with vulval soreness. Vulval colposcopy and directed biopsy confirm vulval intraepithelial neoplasia 1 (VIN I). Discuss the options for her care.

4. A 24-year-old woman has a 2-year history of unexplained infertility. Compare and contrast the management options.

5. What a remarkable impact gonadotrophin releasing hormone analogues (GnRH-a) have made in gynaecology. Review their usage.

Gynaecology answers

1. **A 32-year-old nulliparous woman has long-standing confirmed polycystic ovarian syndrome (PCOS). When attending clinic she states that she intends to stop the combined oral contraceptive pill to conceive. How would you proceed with her care?**

Careful counselling would form the cornerstone of management, involving both the woman and her partner to produce an agreed management plan. A full history would include any history of attempted conception in the past and details regarding the partner. General preconceptual advice regarding folic acid supplementation and cessation of smoking is important. As the incidence of miscarriage is higher in women with polycystic ovarian syndrome (PCOS), particular attention should be paid to other risk factors such as smoking habit in the partner. Weight reduction in the obese will not only improve pregnancy outcome, but may improve the chance of conception in women with PCOS. Secondly, counselling should focus on the possibility of reduced fertility. Expectant management can be adopted for the first 6 months following cessation of the oral contraceptive pill. Follow-up can be arranged for this point, when further discussion can take place. Should the woman experience a regular menstrual cycle of 28 days' duration, ovulation is likely and no action necessary for 1 year. This can be confirmed by the use of day 21 serum progesterone assay or ultrasound follicle tracking. If anovulatory cycles are the predominant pattern, then a carefully monitored 6-month trial of clomiphene would be an appropriate first step. If this is unsuccessful, the couple should proceed to full subfertility investigations prior to any other treatment. This should include a day 2–4 luteinising hormone/follicle stimulating hormone (a prognostic indicator for fertility treatment), rubella and chlamydial screening, semen analysis and a test of tubal patency, the results of which may alter management. In cases of resistant polycystic ovarian syndrome, gonadotrophin induction of ovulation, ovarian diathermy or drilling, or even pulsatile GnRH analogues can be considered. In cases of failed ovulation induction, unexplained infertility or if suggested by the investigations performed, assisted reproduction may be indicated. The risk of ovarian hyperstimulation syndrome is raised in PCOS. If, during treatment, conception does occur, the couple should be seen early following conception to confirm viability and provide reassurance, as miscarriage is a significant risk in women with PCOS.

Comments
This question must be considered in two main parts: (a) preconceptual counselling and (b) applied knowledge of PCOS.
Did you mention the woman's partner?

Suggested reading
Chamberlain G (ed) 1995 Turnbull's obstetrics. Churchill Livingstone, Edinburgh
Franks S 1995 Polycystic ovary syndrome. New England Journal of Medicine 333: 853–861
Hull M G R 1987 Epidemiology of infertility and polycystic ovarian disease: endocrinological and demographic studies. Gynaecological Endocrinology 1: 235–245

2. **Evaluate the range of surgical options available for the treatment of genuine stress incontinence (GSI). On what criteria would you base your selection of an appropriate operation?**

The large array of surgical procedures available for the treatment of genuine stress incontinence reflects the low long-term success rate of incontinence surgery. The suprapubic procedures (Burch colposuspension, Marshall–Marchetti–Krantz or MMK urethropexy, urethrovesical sling) can achieve a success rate of over 80% at 5 years when performed as a primary procedure. However, suprapubic procedures are associated with long-term voiding difficulties (particularly sling procedures) and the increased morbidity of an abdominal incision. The MMK procedure is also associated with osteitis pubis. Laparoscopic colposuspension has lower associated morbidity but appears to have a lower success rate than the open approach. Anterior colporrhaphy also has lower associated morbidity and the need for self-catheterisation is low, but it only achieves a 5-year success rate of around 60% for primary procedures. The success rate of needle suspension (e.g. Stamey) procedures and implants such as collagen is also low. Implantation of an artificial sphincter is a major procedure and unlikely to achieve complete continence, as the pressures required would cause erosion of the urethra. Catheterisation and urinary diversion are available as palliative procedures in cases of repeated surgical failure.

Case selection is vital in the surgical management of GSI. In a healthy younger woman, previous failed surgery, or cases where other pelvic surgery is required, suprapubic surgery is indicated. In repeated surgical failure, a sling procedure would be first choice. Laparoscopic colposuspension may have a place in those women who cannot tolerate the increased morbidity of the open approach or who have cosmetic concerns. Usually, when the patient's age and health will not allow suprapubic surgery, there is a large cystocoele causing discomfort, other vaginal surgery is contemplated or the woman considers the chance of self-catheterisation is unacceptable, an anterior colporrhaphy would be considered. Needle suspension procedures are usually only selected as a primary procedure in elderly women, where vaginal access and capacity are reduced. Implants such as collagen are useful for intrinsic sphincter deficiency, when the bladder neck is well supported.

The success rate is also operator dependent and often influences case selection. Continuing audit, including long-term follow-up, is important.

Comments

The required answer appears to be broad. In a short essay, it is therefore important to group similar techniques (with similar outcomes) together and give one example from each category.

If you are stuck as to where to start with the second part, make a list of difficult operative problems, e.g. the obese patient, previous incontinence surgery, coexistent prolapse, etc. and then demonstrate selection of an appropriate operation according to the problem.

Suggested reading

Jeffcoate T W A, Roberts H 1952 Stress incontinence. British Journal of Obstetrics and Gynaecology 59: 685–720

Nichols D H, Randall C L 1989 Operation for urinary stress incontinence. In: Nichols D H, Randall C L (eds) Vaginal Surgery, 3rd edn. Williams & Wilkins, Baltimore

Royal College of Physicians 1995 Incontinence: cause, management and provision of services. RCP, London

Shaw R W, Soutter W P, Stanton S L (eds) 1996 Gynaecology, 2nd edn. Churchill Livingstone, Edinburgh

3. **All menopausal women should be on hormone replacement therapy (HRT). Critically appraise this statement.**

As the average life expectancy increases in the western world, so the proportion of life spent in the post menopausal state increases. Currently in the United Kingdom, on average, one-third of a woman's life is spent oestrogen deficient. The benefits of HRT are numerous and range from the prevention of osteoporosis and cardiovascular disease to the treatment of symptoms associated with oestrogen decline, e.g. vaginal dryness, skin and hair changes, hot flushes and psychological problems. HRT has even been advocated to slow the progression of Alzheimer's disease. Certainly there are side-effects associated with HRT. There is an increased risk of breast cancer, which may prove to be significant in cases of prolonged HRT administration of over 10 years' duration. A small proportion of women do not tolerate HRT (for example, mastalgia) or are not prepared to tolerate continued menstruation. The advent of new preparations (such as the continuous HRT not requiring a withdrawal bleed) has enabled more women to continue on HRT. However, some women cannot take HRT because of definite contraindications. HRT is absolutely contraindicated in cases of previous or current liver disease, porphyria, unexplained vaginal bleeding, and usually oestrogen-dependent tumours such as endometrial and breast cancer. The advent of selective oestrogen receptor modulator therapy may allow the treatment of some of these women currently denied HRT. In those that can take HRT, the benefits are obvious, leading to improved life expectancy and quality of life. In other countries, the initial expense of providing HRT would be prohibitive, but in the western world, there would be a net cost saving. The reduced incidence of debilitating angina, heart failure and osteoporotic fractures leads to a decreased requirement for social support in the elderly population. Currently, in England, osteoporosis accounts for about £750 000 000 in health care costs per year.

All women cannot take HRT, but all women should be assessed individually and if there are no contraindications, HRT should be offered. Current opinion would suggest that HRT can certainly be taken safely for a period of 10 years.

Comments
The question is on HRT alone, therefore talking about calcium supplements etc. will not gain any points, nor will a review of the different preparations available.

'Critically appraise' implies that the format must be to give a balanced argument including the pros and cons. You may have your own views, but it is prudent to answer in accordance with the general consensus in the current medical press.

Omission of the lay public's fear regarding the increased risk of breast cancer will count heavily against you.

Suggested reading
Ballard P A, Purdie D W 1996 The natural history of osteoporosis. British Journal of Hospital Medicine 55(8): 503–507
Barrett-Connor E 1998 Hormone replacement therapy. British Medical Journal 317: 457–461

4. **A 40-year-old woman is referred by her general practitioner with a single mildly dyskaryotic cervical smear. Critically appraise the options for her care.**

Initially the management choices lie between colposcopic assessment or repeat cytology in 6 months. The majority of patients can safely be managed expectantly. If the repeat smear shows dyskaryosis, then colposcopic assessment would be performed at that point. If the cervical cytology is normal, then a repeat smear in a further 6 months, followed by yearly smears (for 5 years) by the general practitioner should be sufficient. Mild dyskaryosis is a cytological, not histological, diagnosis and so there is a possibility that the pathology is more serious than the cytology would suggest. Therefore, if the woman is symptomatic (intermenstrual or postcoital bleeding) or has a history of abnormal cervical cytology at any time in the past, referral for colposcopic assessment and directed biopsy is advisable. This is also more likely in a woman of 40 years old than in the younger age group. Other risk factors include immunosuppressant therapy and smoking history.

Should colposcopic assessment indicate cervical intraepithelial neoplasia I (CIN I), the case may be managed expectantly if the patient wishes, but many patients opt for active treatment rather than the uncertainty of repeated abnormal smears. In the presence of CIN II/III, treatment is required. Treatment can be performed when directed biopsy results are available, or can be performed at the first visit. The latter 'see and treat' method is cost-effective and preferred by some patients, because of the swiftness of completing definitive treatment. However, treatment can only be carried out at the first visit if the squamocolumnar junction and upper limit of the lesion are well seen and there is no suspicion of malignancy. There can also be a tendency for over-treatment with such a policy. A 'see and treat' policy is better executed by an experienced colposcopist and treatment should be non-destructive. In cases where hysterectomy is being considered for coincidental gynaecological pathology, careful colposcopic assessment and biopsy is essential preoperatively. This colposcopic examination is necessary to exclude more serious changes, for example invasive changes (where a radical hysterectomy would be considered) or the presence of vaginal intraepithelial neoplasia (where a cuff of vagina may need to be taken).

Comments

Most referral protocols require a second abnormal smear prior to colposcopic referral. But this question is not asking for a regurgitation of your local protocol. Think carefully: is this always the case?

The question omits whether this woman has a history of smear abnormality, has had abnormal bleeding or whether there are other gynaecological problems.

When seen in colposcopy, the discussion should focus on the merits of a 'see and treat' policy versus 'treat after results'.

Suggested reading

Bigrigg A, Browning J 1993 The treatment of cervical intraepithelial neoplasia. In: Studd J (ed) Progress in obstetrics and gynaecology. Churchill Livingstone, Edinburgh, vol 10, pp 359–375

Campion M J, McCane D J, Cuzik J, Singer A 1986 Progressive potential of mild cervical atypia: prospective cytological, colposcopic and virological study. Lancet ii: 237–240

Robertson J H, Wooden B E, Crozier E H, Hutchinson J 1988 Risk of cervical cancer associated with mild dyskaryosis. British Medical Journal 297(2): 18–21

5. **At 9 weeks and after slight vaginal bleeding, an ultrasound scan confirms the presence of a missed abortion. Compare and contrast possible courses of action.**

There are three main options in this case. Careful and thorough counselling is required to determine the patient's preference, as this is the dominant influence on the choice taken. The first option is to await spontaneous miscarriage. This has the disadvantage that a surgical evacuation will still probably be required and there is an increased risk of infection and haemorrhage with this approach. Some couples prefer this, however, owing to religious objections. Others find it easier psychologically to leave the decision to nature. Rescanning in a week, should miscarriage not intervene, allows some couples to accept that the pregnancy is non-viable.

If intervention is chosen, evacuation of the uterus can be a medical or a surgical procedure. Surgical evacuation of the uterus currently comprises 75% of the emergency gynaecological operations. In the case of a missed abortion, an evacuation would not be a purely surgical procedure, as (unless contraindicated) a dose of intravaginal gemeprost should be given preoperatively to reduce the chance of cervical trauma. Medical evacuation involves the usage of mifepristone, followed 36–48 hours later by gemeprost 1 mg vaginally. Medical evacuations have several advantages over surgical evacuation. Medical evacuation avoids the usage of routine and emergency operating time. The woman avoids the risks of a general anaesthetic, cervical trauma, uterine perforation and intrauterine adhesions associated with a surgical evacuation. This approach is usually more cost-effective. However, some women find the procedure distressing, particularly if an emergency evacuation is required anyway, such as in cases of heavy bleeding. This procedure is contraindicated in cases of cardiac disease and asthma and there is a risk of anaphylaxis. Some women experience significant pain and require opiate analgesia, whilst others experience nausea, vomiting and diarrhoea. Medical evacuation requires a completely different care package and therefore this may be difficult to cater for on a traditional gynaecology ward. There is limited information on the management preference of women with a blighted ovum. There is evidence that, rather than there being an optimum management pathway, patients highly value the availability of choice.

Comments
The question asked for possible courses of action to be compared and contrasted. This essay type means that a clear account of the pros and cons of all options is required. The emphasis is not on justifying one particular course of action.

The central concept is that of the woman's preference being the main determinant of management.

Suggested reading
Chipchase J, James D 1997 Randomised trial of expectant versus surgical management of spontaneous miscarriage. British Journal of Obstetrics and Gynaecology 104: 840–841

Henshaw R C, Templeton A A 1993 Antiprogesterones. In: Progress in obstetrics and gynaecology, vol 10. Churchill Livingstone, Edinburgh, pp 259–279

Howie F L 1997 Medical abortion or vacuum aspiration? Two year follow-up of a patient preference trial. British Journal of Obstetrics and Gynaecology 104: 829–833

PAPER 2

1. Review the recent advances and probable future developments in contraception.

There is continuous development of the choice of contraception for both male and female, fuelled by the dissatisfaction of many couples with the current options. The long established natural methods of contraception (the only methods acceptable to some religious groups) have recently been refined by the introduction of home urinary luteinising hormone (LH) monitoring ('Persona'). In some series of well-motivated couples, it has achieved a Pearl Index (number of pregnancies per 100 woman years) of 6. Barrier contraception has seen the introduction of a wide range of condoms (e.g. polymer), spermicides and the female condom. The last has not achieved a sufficient level of patient acceptability. The combined oral contraceptive pill remains a safe and popular option, despite adverse publicity. The introduction of even lower dosage regimes, alternative progestogens and the possible use of mifepristone should lead to still further advances in safety and acceptability. As progesterone-only preparations are known to have a particularly low incidence of cardiovascular and thromboembolic complications, long-acting versions using levonorgestrel have been developed. The subcutaneous implant (e.g. Norplant: 5 years' duration) and the intrauterine contraceptive device (e.g. Mirena: 3 years' duration) appear to be as effective as sterilisation (0.14 for Mirena, 0–0.5 for female sterilisation). Unlike sterilisation, however, these preparations are rapidly reversible.

The advent of open laparoscopy may result in more women being suitable for sterilisation as a day case procedure.

Improvements in emergency contraception (Yuzpe regime prevents only 80–90% of expected pregnancies) may be made by the usage of mifepristone (RU486). One of the most promising areas of research includes immunocontraception. The basis of this approach is that the vaccine blocks a vital part of the reproductive pathway, for example the action of beta hCG. One side-effect may well be the suppression of the ovary. Exogenous testosterone has been disappointing to date, but this immunological approach may yet yield an effective male contraceptive.

Comments

The question addresses the recent advances and probable future developments in contraception. This needs wide knowledge of the current methods, recent advances and what is expected from developing research; *but* this question did *not* ask for a review of all methods of contraception.

There will definitely be a question on family planning in the examination, if not in the written paper, then in the RCOG oral assessment examination. Revision of contraception should be a top priority!

As with a question on subfertility, you must remember that it is an issue for both male and female.

More points will be gained with this broad question if an overview is given rather than concentrating in great detail on one aspect. Giving an example from each category of contraception (barrier, hormonal, IUCD, etc.) is better than writing an entire essay on the advances in the make-up of the combined oral contraception pill.

Suggested reading
Guillebaud J 1995 Advising women on which pill to take. British Medical
    Journal 311: 1111–1112
Loudon N, Glossier A, Gebbie A 1995 Handbook of family planning,
    3rd edn. Churchill Livingstone, Edinburgh
Tayob Y, Guillebaud J 1990 Barrier methods of contraception. In: Studd
    J (ed) Progress in obstetrics and gynaecology. Churchill Livingstone,
    Edinburgh, vol 8, pp 371–390

2. **A 24-year-old woman has persistent vaginal bleeding following a dilatation and curettage for gestational trophoblastic tumour (GTT). Give a detailed account of your management.**

The time interval must be established in relation to the operation. In the immediate postoperative period, perforation of the uterus, retained products and the existence of an invasive mole or even choriocarcinoma must be considered. The degree of blood loss and cardiovascular status of the patient should govern management. If the bleeding is heavy or does not settle, re-evacuation of the uterus, accompanied by laparoscopy to exclude perforation, is indicated following adequate resuscitation. Recourse to hysterectomy may be required. Anti D must be administered to rhesus-negative women.

In later presentations, a differential diagnosis would include infection, retained molar tissue, or a further pregnancy. Retained molar tissue is common, as there may be an element of myometrial invasion. The availability of histological information should help to exclude choriocarcinoma. Evidence of metastasis should be sought, including chest examination and chest X-ray. The risk of choriocarcinoma is higher in blood group B and AB women, particularly if the partner's blood group differs. Malaise, lower abdominal pain and offensive discharge suggest infection: a higher vaginal swab should be taken and antibiotics given. A bulky, tender uterus and an open cervical os on pelvic examination suggest retained products of conception, as does continued bleeding following treatment of an intrauterine infection. Blood should be taken for full blood count, group and save and quantitative serum beta human chorionic gonadotrophin (beta hCG). A beta hCG rise and an ultrasound scan examination (preferably transvaginal) will diagnose a further pregnancy or residual trophoblastic disease. Uterine re-evacuation must be performed by an experienced operator, owing to the increased risk of uterine perforation. Long-term follow-up is coordinated via one of the three UK reference laboratories, initially utilising serum beta hCG and later urinary hCG estimation. If the bleeding settles and the hCG drops to undetectable levels, barrier contraception can be converted to the combined oral contraceptive and the patient can be advised that she can retry for a pregnancy after a year. Recurrence of vaginal bleeding or failure of the hCG levels to drop to normal suggests the necessity for referral to one of the specialist centres for chemotherapy.

Comments
The question omits the time scale and the severity of the blood loss. Do not approach this question with tunnel vision. You need to discuss management of this postoperative complication of a D&C as well as discussing the particular risks associated with GTT.

The examiners are obviously looking for a demonstration that you can manage this gynaecological emergency safely: (a) resuscitation first; (b) the need for an experienced surgeon; and (c) showing that you recognise the increased risk of perforation of the uterus and retained products of conception and the possibility of choriocarcinoma.

Suggested reading
Chamberlain G (ed) 1995 Turnbull's obstetrics. Churchill Livingstone, Edinburgh
Newlands E S 1995 Clinical management of trophoblastic disease in the UK. Current Obstetrics and Gynaecology 5: 19–24

3. **Following a total abdominal hysterectomy and bilateral salpingo-oophorectomy for endometriosis, a 39-year-old woman presents with continuous urinary incontinence. How would you assess this problem?**

A total abdominal hysterectomy for endometriosis can be difficult and the concern here would be that unrecognised intraoperative bladder or ureteric damage may have resulted in fistula formation. This is also suggested by the continuous nature of the urinary loss. Other possibilities include severe detrusor instability or gross stress incontinence. Assessment would primarily take the form of a detailed history and examination. The woman may volunteer a history of incontinence predating the operation. A detailed review of the notes is required. The operation note may indicate that the procedure was difficult and that there was a possibility of urinary tract injury at the time. Haematuria followed by immediate incontinence postoperatively would suggest direct injury to the urinary tract. Partial-thickness damage to the bladder, for example by excessive diathermy or devascularisation of the lower ureter presents later, the incontinence starting 7–14 days postoperatively. On vaginal examination, a pool of urine may be visible in the vagina or the fistula itself may be visible. On coughing, obvious leakage from the urethra would suggest stress incontinence. If the urinary leakage is in doubt, a pad test can be applied. A vesicovaginal fistula may be demonstrated by a three swab test. Three swabs are placed in the vagina and diluted methylene blue instilled into the bladder via a urethral catheter. Staining of the swabs in the upper vagina suggests a vesicovaginal fistula but not a ureterovaginal fistula. An intravenous urogram and cystogram will demonstrate conclusively a ureterovaginal fistula and a vesicovaginal fistula. Further assessment by examination under anaesthesia, including cystoscopy, is essential prior to planning reconstructive surgery. The team who will be repairing the fistula preferably should perform this assessment. Fistula repair may require multidisciplinary input.

Where a fistula has been excluded, investigations for detrusor instability may be helpful. Detrusor instability is a recognised postoperative complication following hysterectomy. A frequency volume chart may suggest detrusor instability. Urodynamic assessment by cystometry will differentiate detrusor instability and genuine stress incontinence. Where there are equivocal results, improvement following an empirical trial of oxybutynin would support the diagnosis of detrusor instability.

Comments

The question asks for assessment of the problem. This includes clinical methods as well as appropriate investigations. The time scale involved and details regarding the preoperative urinary history have been omitted.

Recognition of the possibility of a fistula is a very important point demonstrating safe practice, so remember to put it first! Remember to mention the value of multidisciplinary input, as it crosses the speciality boundary.

Suggested reading

Rock J A 1995 Endometriosis: critical developments in understanding and management. International Journal of Gynaecology and Obstetrics 50(suppl 1): 1–42

Shaw R W 1991 Treatment of endometriosis. In: Studd J (ed) Progress in obstetrics and gynaecology. Churchill Livingstone, Edinburgh, vol 9, pp 273–287

Tindall V R 1990 Jeffcoate's principles of gynaecology, 5th edn. Butterworths, London

4. **A 35-year-old woman presents with amenorrhoea and vasomotor symptoms. Subsequent serum follicle stimulating hormone (FSH) and luteinising hormone (LH) levels are markedly raised. Explore further management.**

This clinical picture associated with markedly raised FSH and LH is diagnostic of premature menopause. Careful exploration of the history may reveal a family history of premature menopause, as the most common cause is familial. In others, there may be risk factors such as preceding serious illness, radiotherapy or chemotherapy. Chromosomal abnormalities (e.g. Turner's mosaic) are also associated and therefore karyotyping is justified.

Premature menopause can have a devastating effect and careful counselling is essential. There are two main areas of concern: the long-term health risks posed by oestrogen deficiency and the impact of the premature end to reproductive life. The most important long-term health risks are those of cardiovascular disease and osteoporosis. A baseline bone scan is useful. Long-term compliance to hormone replacement therapy (HRT) is essential. Care must be taken to select a method of administration which is acceptable to the woman. In order to achieve symptom control in such a young woman, the higher-dose regimes will be required (e.g. oestradiol valerate 2 mg). Infertility is not guaranteed and contraception should be continued for 2 years. The low-dose combined oral contraceptive pill is appropriate to fulfil both roles, HRT and contraception, during this period. Some women will be devastated as they are unlikely to be able to conceive. This is an increasingly important issue as more women delay pregnancy until their 30s. The options can be explored with the woman and her partner: In vitro fertilisation (IVF) with oocyte donation, surrogacy or adoption. If assisted reproduction is the chosen route, infertility investigation of both the woman and her partner must be accomplished quickly. As the waiting lists for IVF are long and oocyte donors scarce, prompt referral to a specialist centre for assisted reproduction is required.

Comments
The question omits parity: a clue that infertility may be an important issue.
   Did you mention the partner?
   Issues such as adoption and surrogacy need to be mentioned.

Suggested reading
Anasti J N 1998 Premature ovarian failure: an update. Fertility and
   Sterility 70: 1–15
Baber R, Abdalla H, Studd J 1991 The premature menopause. In: Studd
   J (ed) Progress in obstetrics and gynaecology. Churchill Livingstone,
   Edinburgh, vol 9, pp 209–226
Nilsson P 1997 Social and biological predictors of early menopause: a
   model for premature aging. Journal of Internal Medicine 242: 299–305

5. **How would you construct and implement a unit policy for thromboembolic prophylaxis for gynaecological surgery?**

The presence of an effective protocol for thromboembolic prophylaxis in gynaecological surgery is of major importance, as highlighted by the RCOG Working Party 1995. The National Confidential Enquiry into Perioperative Deaths (CEPOD) (DoH 1993) indicates that fatal thromboembolism is responsible for around 20% of deaths associated with hysterectomy. An effective protocol can only be devised with the participation and motivation of all staff involved. This involves not only gynaecologists and anaesthetists, but also ward and theatre staff, nurses, technicians and physiotherapists. Essential to the introduction of such a system is the co-introduction of an efficient audit. The current practice and patient outcome should be initially audited. A risk-assessment profile must be devised for each patient, based on history, examination and procedure to be undertaken, designating the woman as either low, medium or high risk. Major surgery, older patients, obesity, smoking, family history or personal history of thromboembolism, intercurrent medical illness (e.g. heart disease) or infection, preoperative immobility and malignancy (particularly gynaecological malignancy) are all risk factors for thromboembolism. In low-risk cases and those undergoing minor surgery, early mobilisation and the avoidance of dehydration is all that is required. In those patients of moderate risk, a mechanical method of prophylaxis should be added, such as pneumatic calf compression or graduated elastic stockings. High-risk cases require a mechanical method of prophylaxis, early mobilisation and exercises from the physiotherapist and heparin prophylaxis. Other methods which can be considered include dextran 70 and aspirin, but these are less commonly used. Following the introduction of the protocol, a further audit should be performed to close the audit loop. In this way, the protocol can be continuously updated and improved.

Comments

The candidate must demonstrate an awareness of the current problem, the construction of protocols and the intrinsic importance of audit.

A knowledge of the 'take-home' messages of CEPOD (Confidential Enquiry into Perioperative Deaths) can be utilised to good effect in this type of question.

Write an essay plan for the equivalent essay in obstetrics.

Suggested reading

Chamberlain G (ed) 1995 Turnbull's obstetrics. Churchill Livingstone, Edinburgh

Department of Health 1993 Report of the National Confidential Enquiry into Perioperative Deaths 1991/1992. HMSO, London

Nelson-Piercy C 1996 Obstetric prophylaxis. British Journal of Hospital Medicine 55(7): 404–407

Royal College of Obstetricians and Gynaecologists 1995 Report of the RCOG Working Party on Prophylaxis Against Thromboembolism in Gynaecology and Obstetrics. RCOG, London

PAPER 3

1. **Critically evaluate the current controversies in the field of assisted reproduction.**

The development of assisted reproduction has been followed by controversy since its beginning. On the one hand, it is embraced by the 1 in 10 couples who are affected by subfertility. On the other hand, there are substantial religious and moral objections to these revolutionary techniques. As an attempt to address these issues, assisted reproduction in the UK is regulated and guided by HFEA (Human Fertilisation and Embryology Authority). In particular, techniques involving ovum, sperm and gamete donation have special problems. There are questions regarding the offspring's rights regarding their genetic parents and yet donors must be afforded protection. The recent case regarding the claim of a widow to use her late husband's semen has highlighted the legal uncertainty of 'ownership' of stored semen and gametes. Legislation requires constant review, as unforeseen ethical dilemmas occur frequently in this uncharted field. An example has been the recent concern regarding the 5-year limit to the storage of embryos. This was extended, provided both genetic parents gave consent. This proved difficult where one genetic parent was a donor. Recent publicity has also surrounded surrogacy, demonstrating the emotional aspects as well as questioning the morality of financial payments and the implications for child welfare. Child welfare is a central concern regarding the selection of women for treatment, highlighted by the cases of successful conception in women over 50 years of age. Other examples which are a source of controversy include preimplantation testing, selective fetocide and research involving embryos. Assisted reproduction is a technologically demanding treatment and as such is expensive. Despite this, the 'take home baby rate' is low overall. The major debate in the National Health Service is that of appropriateness of funding such a service in these days of scarce resources.

Comments

Awareness of practice in the UK is essential to answer this question. Information is usually gathered from the media rather than textbooks. So talk about these issues to a consultant who has an interest in subfertility. Keep up to date with the broadsheet newspapers, *Hospital Doctor* and read the news pages and editorials of the *BMJ*, *Lancet* and the *British Journal of Obstetrics and Gynaecology.*

   HFEA must be mentioned, as it is the body that governs the practice of assisted conception in the UK.

Suggested reading

Abdalla H, Baber R, Studd J 1990 Active management of infertility. In: Studd J (ed) Progress in obstetrics and gynaecology. Churchill Livingstone, Edinburgh, vol 8, pp 273–287

Brazier M, Golombok S, Campbell A 1997 Surrogacy: review for the UK Health Ministers of current arrangements for payments and regulation. Human Reproductive Update 623–628

Craft N 1996 BMA issues new guidance on surrogacy (news). British Medical Journal 312: 397–398

2. **A 19-year-old woman presents with lower abdominal pain associated with vaginal discharge, both of 8 days' duration. Because of worsening pain and a pyrexia, her general practitioner has sought a gynaecological opinion. How would you proceed with her care?**

This is a common presentation encountered as a gynaecological emergency. Full evaluation of the patient by taking a history and performing a clinical examination, including a pelvic examination, is essential. In particular, the nature and site of the pain, contraceptive history including the intrauterine contraceptive device (IUCD), menstrual, sexual history and details of any previous episodes should be ascertained. Examination should focus on the site of the pain, the presence of any masses and the amount and nature of the discharge. From this picture, pelvic inflammatory disease is the most likely diagnosis and would be supported by bilateral tenderness in the adnexae. Swabs must be taken: a high vaginal swab, endocervical swab (for gonococcus) and an endocervical chlamydial swab. The woman should be counselled and the IUCD removed if present and sent for culture. Dependent on the sexual history, rectal and urethral swabs may be appropriate. A full blood count must be performed in view of the pyrexia. In the case of a high pyrexia, blood cultures should be considered. A pregnancy test should be performed as a routine in all women with acute lower abdominal pain, in case of an atypical presentation of an ectopic pregnancy, even though the diagnosis appears clear cut in this case. Ultrasound scan examination may be of value if a pelvic collection or pyosalpinx is suspected. The woman should be admitted and intravenous antibiotics should be commenced and maintained for 48 hours. These should be broad spectrum, such as a cephalosporin and metronidazole and the regime should also incorporate an antibiotic that covers chlamydia (such as doxycycline). This should be taken for a minimum of 10 days. Should improvement not occur within 24 hours, the diagnosis should be reappraised. A diagnostic laparoscopy is indicated to establish a diagnosis and a surgical opinion considered. Early and effective treatment of pelvic inflammatory disease is of paramount importance to reduce the long-term sequelae of pelvic pain, subfertility and ectopic pregnancy. In addition, consideration should be given to referral to genitourinary medicine for a full screen for sexually transmitted diseases and tracing of sexual contacts.

Comments
This is a typical gynaecological emergency, testing the basic knowledge of a trainee. The question asks for a comprehensive answer covering history, examination, investigation, treatment and follow-up.

Note that, in this question, the actual diagnosis is omitted. Therefore, although your answer must mainly concern pelvic inflammatory disease, you must discuss the important differential diagnoses, particularly the possibility of ectopic pregnancy.

There are different schools of thought regarding the diagnosis of pelvic inflammatory disease. Some people believe that laparoscopy is essential to establish the diagnosis, but it is practical to start treatment immediately and then to carry out a diagnostic laparoscopy if no improvement in the woman's general condition has occurred after 24 hours' observation.

Suggested reading

Benaim J, Pulaski M, Coupey S M 1998 Adolescent girls and pelvic inflammatory disease. Archives of Paediatrics and Adolescent Medicine 152: 449–454

Blythe M J 1998 Pelvic inflammatory disease in the adolescent population. Seminars in Paediatric Surgery 7: 43–51

Centers for Disease Control and Prevention 1991 Pelvic inflammatory disease: guidelines for prevention and management. Morbidity and Mortality Weekly Report 40(RR-5): 1–25. CDC, Atlanta

Stacey C M, Barton S E, Singer A 1991 Pelvic inflammatory disease. In : Studd J (ed) Progress in obstetrics and gynaecology. Churchill Livingstone, Edinburgh, vol 9, pp 259–271

3. A 17-year-old girl presents with primary amenorrhoea. How would you reach a diagnosis?

It is very important that the clinician has a clear methodical approach to investigate this problem, as the pathway to reaching a diagnosis can be complicated. Reaching a diagnosis will depend on the differential diagnosis of primary amenorrhoea and this depends on the history, examination and relevant investigations. The history should include developmental history and family history of any sisters and mother. Examination will include general examination, looking at the patient's build, and local examination, particularly looking at secondary sexual characteristics (including breast development and the distribution of hair). The investigations may include a pregnancy test (pregnancy should be excluded if she is sexually active), Follicle stimulating hormone (FSH), luteinising hormone (LH), serum prolactin, blood for chromosomal analysis, thyroid function tests and a scan of the uterus and ovaries. A progestogen challenge test may be carried out, giving medroxyprogesterone acetate 5 mg daily for 5 days to check endogenous oestrogen levels. The appearance of withdrawal bleeding shows that the endometrium is reactive and the outflow tract patent. If the prolactin level is significantly high, a pituitary tumour must be excluded by performing a CT scan. If, after the progestogen challenge test, no bleeding occurs, it is essential to have the FSH and LH levels. If LH is low, this may suggest hypogonadotrophic hypogonadism. A high FSH, more than 40 IU/L on successive readings, indicates ovarian failure. If this is the case, karyotyping would be essential in view of the suspicion of Turner's syndrome. On the other hand, a low FSH and LH of less than 3 IU/L suggests constitutionally delayed puberty or hypothalamic amenorrhoea. A raised LH of more than 10 IU/L and a normal FSH suggests polycystic ovarian syndrome.

Comments

Did you read the question? The question asks 'How would you reach a diagnosis?'. The answer should not be restricted to information on investigations, but must mention history and examination in addition. Talking about other management issues, however, will waste time and space and not gain any extra marks!

The answer requires a clear investigative pathway to be described, not just a list of investigations. The examiner will be interested in your logic, not just your factual knowledge.

Pregnancy should be excluded in all cases of amenorrhoea, whether it is primary or secondary.

Suggested reading
Edmonds D K 1993 Primary amenorrhoea. In: Studd J (ed) Progress in obstetrics and gynaecology. Churchill Livingstone, Edinburgh, vol 10, pp 281–295

4. Evaluate the place of laparoscopy in current gynaecological practice.

With the technological advances in fibreoptics, this has become an essential tool in both gynaecological diagnosis and minimal-access surgery. Diagnostic laparoscopy has a wide range of applications and has become indispensable to the gynaecologist. For diagnostic procedures, laparoscopy can be used in acute gynaecological problems, such as establishing the diagnosis of pelvic inflammatory disease, ovarian cysts (and attendant complications) and ectopic pregnancies. These are by far the commonest gynaecological problems addressed by laparoscopy. Chronic conditions such as endometriosis and recurrent pelvic pain due to a congested pelvis are also diagnosed with laparoscopy. Missing coils, following perforation of the uterus, can be visualised with the aid of laparoscopy and cases of polycystic disease can be detected.

Operative laparoscopy has developed rapidly. Laparoscopic sterilisation is by far the commonest laparoscopic procedure performed. Simple ovarian cysts can be aspirated or deroofed and salpingectomy or conservative surgery for ectopic pregnancy performed laparoscopically. Endometriosis can be destroyed with diathermy or laser, with the aid of the laparoscope under direct vision, and resistant polycystic ovarian disease can be treated laparoscopically by ovarian diathermy or laser drilling. Although oocyte aspiration is largely now accomplished under ultrasound guidance, laparoscopic tubal surgery and gamete intrafallopian transfer (GIFT) have established laparoscopic surgery in a central role. Laparoscopically assisted vaginal hysterectomy seems to have found a place in current gynaecological practice. However, laparoscopic hysterectomy and myomectomy have not achieved the popularity expected, owing to a relatively high incidence of complications and long operative time, in an atmosphere of increasing medical litigation.

Overall, operative laparoscopy has a significant advantage, as the recovery time following laparoscopic procedures is far less than after open procedures because, in the absence of complications, patient morbidity is reduced. The resulting reduction in hospital stay produces a significant financial saving for health authorities, even after the increased operating time has been taken into account. On the other hand, laparoscopic techniques can be implicated in significant complications such as ureteric injury, haemorrhage and bowel trauma, culminating in serious patient morbidity. The greatest risk factor for this is laparoscopic techniques being used by inadequately trained individuals.

Comments
The question is to evaluate the place of laparoscopy in gynaecological practice. The answer is not restricted to laparoscopic surgery. Did you split down your answer into diagnostic and therapeutic?

Note the key word 'evaluate', therefore the answer is not just restricted to a description of the role of laparoscopy, but must include some assessment of its value.

Suggested reading
Tindall V R 1990 Jeffcoate's principles of gynaecology, 5th edn. Butterworths, London

5. **A 47-year-old woman has a hysterectomy due to intractable menorrhagia. The subsequent histology report reads as follows: 'Uterus: within the cavity of the uterus is a well differentiated adenocarcinoma. This tumour infiltrates the myometrium, but this is superficial, being confined to the inner one-third of the myometrium'. How would you conduct her subsequent care?**

Such a case poses several clinical dilemmas. According to FIGO (International Federation of Obstetrics and Gynaecology) recommendations, the management of endometrial carcinoma depends on accurate surgical staging. As this pathology was not suspected preoperatively, the ovaries may have been conserved and lymph node sampling omitted. The woman should be assessed on an individual basis, taking into account her relatively young age and general health. It must be borne in mind that the patient is completely unprepared for the histological findings and she must be counselled carefully regarding the options available. The options to be considered include no further action, further surgery or radiotherapy. In expectant management, computerised tomography or magnetic resonance imaging can be utilised to assess the likelihood of lymphatic spread, but this is not as effective as surgical staging. Adopting a surgical approach would also allow bilateral oophorectomy to be performed if required, as well as formal surgical staging to be completed. Although the incidence of metastasis to the ovaries is low, conservation of the ovaries may lead to rapid progression of any residual tumour, owing to its oestrogen-dependent nature. This approach carries the risks of further surgery, including wound infection and thromboembolism and would be of particular concern in a woman with intercurrent medical problems. The third option would be to offer external beam radiotherapy. Radiotherapy treats metastatic spread as well as producing a radiation menopause where the ovaries have been conserved. However, the disadvantages of radiotherapy are not restricted to the short-term side-effects of cystitis and gastrointestinal disturbance, but also the long-term sequelae of bowel strictures, fistula formation and importantly in this relatively young woman, vaginal stenosis. Realistically, in view of the well-differentiated nature, superficial invasion and confinement to the body of the uterus of this tumour, the chance of metastasis is low. This, in conjunction with the increased morbidity posed by radiotherapy or further surgery, means that where the ovaries have been removed, further intervention is probably not justified. Adjuvant therapy with progesterone can be considered. As endometrial carcinoma is oestrogen dependent, hormone replacement therapy is not usually given.

Comments
Don't get so involved in the oncological details that you miss obvious clinical points.

This is not a straightforward question on the postoperative management of endometrial carcinoma. This was unexpected and therefore a shock to both patient and surgeon. Patient counselling is obviously important. If the surgeon had known, would he have operated differently and, if so, can it be corrected now?

A histology report could also form the basis of a new RCOG oral assessment examination station, as could a cervical cytology report. Look through the histology results on your unit and practise discussing them with another candidate.

Suggested reading
Lawton F G 1993 Early endometrial carcinoma: no more 'TAH, BSO and cuff'. In: Studd J (ed) Progress in obstetrics and gynaecology. Churchill Livingstone, Edinburgh, vol 10, pp 403–413

PAPER 4

1. All gynaecological malignancies should be treated in specialised centres. Critically appraise this statement.

This has been an active area of debate in recent times. The Department of Health document, 'A policy framework for commissioning cancer services' (DoH 1995) suggested that all cancer cases be treated in designated centres, to allow all patients access to a uniformly high standard of care. The focusing of care for gynae-oncology into gynaecological oncology centres has many advantages. Concentration of resources provides significant cost saving. Good quality treatment is facilitated as the patient would be dealt with by a subspecialist in the field, supported by specialist radiologists, nurses, technicians, pain control anaesthetists and gynaepathologists. It would allow concentration of experience, allowing rarer tumours to be treated appropriately. The higher throughput would provide improved training for subspeciality trainees and the increased facilities would provide opportunity for a coherent follow-up structure and data collection system, which can create the basis for future research and development. However, gynaecological malignancies account for a considerable percentage of all malignancies in females (14 000–15 000 cases per annum in the UK) and as such produce a significant workload. Unless such a centre was carefully planned and fully resourced, there is every possibility that the centre could be overwhelmed. Shifting oncological work away from the generalist could have a detrimental effect on standard gynaecological training, resulting in trainees seeing an inadequate number of gynae-oncology cases. Treatment in a specialised centre distant from home places additional stress on the patient. The patient and her family have to cope with transport difficulties and this could present financial problems. The woman may have to cope with being apart from friends and family and their support and this can cause significant family disruption. There are also financial implications for health authorities transferring patients. Treatment in specialised centres may be the way forward in improving standards in the treatment of gynaecological cancer, but there are many practical problems to be addressed. Such a centre is best suited to those areas of high population density. Other areas, where greater travelling distances are involved, may benefit by the maintenance of satellite centres served by outreach clinics and governed by strict management protocols.

Comments

The question is looking for a balanced argument: the advantages and disadvantages of such a policy. If totally unprepared, you may still produce an adequate answer by the application of a little common sense. Think in terms of the implications for the patients, their relatives and the staff involved. Remember to consider training implications, cost-effectiveness, research and audit.

Suggested reading

Department of Health 1995 A policy framework for commissioning cancer services. Guidance for purchasers and providers of cancer services. HMSO, London

Junor E J, Hole D J, Gillis C R 1994 Management of ovarian cancer: referral to a multidisciplinary team matters. British Journal of Cancer 70: 363–370

Kehoe S, Powell J, Wilson S et al 1994 The influence of the operation surgeon's specialisation on patient survival in ovarian cancer. British Journal of Cancer 70: 1014–1017

Kitchener H 1997 Gynaecological cancer services: time for change. British Journal of Obstetrics and Gynaecology 104: 123–126

Woodman C 1997 What changes in the organisation of cancer services will improve the outcome for women with ovarian cancer? British Journal of Obstetrics and Gynaecology 104: 135–139

2. An 11-year-old girl presents with vaginal bleeding following a fall. How would you approach her care?

The first priority would be to quantify the blood loss and assess the girl's clinical condition. If the bleeding is heavy, the next priority should be to establish intravenous access, take bloods for a full blood count and blood cross-match and commence resuscitation. A full history must be taken and include the timing and mechanism of injury, possibility of a penetrating injury and nature of other injuries. The ability to pass urine following the injury is important, as urinary retention is common. Details regarding menarche should be taken and the possibility of a coincidental cause remembered (for example menses, pathology such as the rare sarcoma botryoides or even pregnancy). In any case of genital injury to a child, it is important to consider child abuse if there are any inconsistencies in the history or examination. Early involvement of the paediatric team in any possible case of child abuse is mandatory. Examination should take place with both the mother and a nurse chaperone present. A full general examination should look for other injuries sustained during the fall or suggestive of child abuse. Genital examination should be limited to external inspection of the vulva and introitus, looking particularly for lacerations or active bleeding from the vulva or introitus. In the absence of a penetrating injury or active bleeding, no further action is required. If there are minor labial lacerations which are not actively bleeding, these can usually be managed conservatively. Advice can be given regarding micturition in the bath, if there is difficulty in passing urine. Occasionally, 24–48 hours of urinary catheterisation is required with significant lacerations or bruising. If there is active bleeding from the vagina, a penetrating injury, or there are labial lacerations requiring repair, vaginal examination and suturing under general anaesthesia is required. This should be performed by an experienced gynaecologist, as examination of the vagina and access can be difficult in a girl of this age and for medicolegal reasons. Careful examination of the vagina may require an endoscopic approach or the usage of a head light and a small speculum (possibly a nasal speculum) or paediatric laryngoscope.

Comments

Paediatric gynaecology is an important part of modern gynaecology. Handling of these cases needs senior involvement and detailed explanation to parents. There are a few important principles that the candidate should show awareness of when answering a question on paediatric gynaecology. Keep a checklist: Is there a possibility of abuse? History and examination must always be performed with the mother and preferably with an experienced nurse chaperone present. Internal examination must always be performed under a general anaesthetic. The per rectal approach may be more appropriate for bimanual examination. An experienced gynaecologist must be involved.

Note the age. It has been deliberately picked so that coincidental menarche is a possibility.

Suggested reading
Shaw R W, Soutter W P, Stanton S L (eds) 1996 Gynaecology, 2nd edn. Churchill Livingstone, Edinburgh

Tindall V R 1990 Jeffcoate's principles of gynaecology, 5th edn. Butterworths, London

3. **A 50-year-old lady presents with a 2-year history of worsening stress and urge incontinence. Consider the options for further investigation of this problem.**

A detailed history and examination determine the pattern of investigation, with the aim of assessing the severity and finding the cause of incontinence. As oestrogen deficiency has a detrimental effect on bladder function, a serum luteinising hormone (LH) and follicle stimulating hormone (FSH) assay may be justified. A midstream specimen of urine is required in cases of recurrent cystitis or significant urinary frequency. The simple, non-invasive pad test (the woman performs a variety of activities whilst wearing a pad) is limited to providing more objective quantification of incontinence. A frequency volume chart allows a more objective analysis of symptoms. Suspicion of detrusor instability can be raised by the presence of marked frequency, varying voided volumes and nocturia. A flow rate is of limited use, except to determine if voiding is normal prior to surgery. It can be misleading, unless combined with pressure monitoring, and is therefore best performed at the time of cystometry. Cystometry forms the basis of the diagnostic tests for genuine stress incontinence and detrusor instability, but it is costly, time-consuming, invasive and has a significant number of false negative results for detrusor instability. Simple cystometry has been criticised as being non-physiological and ambulatory urodynamics advocated. This has a higher pick-up for phasic instability, but is prone to artefact, difficult to interpret and requires complex, expensive equipment. Video urodynamics, where cystometry is supplemented by radiological contrast studies, provides anatomical information and is considered to be the gold standard of urodynamic investigation. This would be indicated if there is a suggestion of ureteric reflux, neurological dysfunction, previous surgery or if other studies have been inconclusive. However, this study has the added drawback of radiation exposure. Vaginal ultrasound has been suggested as being a reliable screening test for detrusor instability (measurement of the bladder base being more than 5 mm). Urethral pressure profiles (UPP) are advocated by some authorities, as a low UPP indicates poor surgical outcome, but this is still largely regarded as a research tool. Cystoscopy would be indicated if this woman has haematuria, a small bladder capacity and a hypersensitive or poorly compliant bladder.

Comments

It is important that you make it clear that investigation is mandatory prior to surgery with this clinical picture and that video urodynamics is currently considered to be the gold standard.

It is equally important to discuss *all* the options for investigation and discuss the rationale behind each choice.

It is important that past incontinence surgery must be mentioned as this is a common management problem in incontinence.

Remember, there are no points for straying outside investigations into other management issues.

Suggested reading

Chapple C R, Christmas T J (eds) 1990 Urodynamics made easy. Churchill Livingstone, Edinburgh

Mundy A R, Stephenson T P, Wein A J 1994 Urodynamics: principles, practice and application, 2nd edn. Churchill Livingstone, Edinburgh

4. **A 32-year-old woman presents with primary infertility. A laparoscopic survey reveals endometriosis. Critically evaluate the management options.**

Management of this woman and her partner will depend on the history and examination findings, as well as laparoscopy and investigation results. Careful counselling regarding treatment options is essential. The benefits of treatment of endometriosis must be balanced against time lost in commencing fertility treatment. The success of fertility treatment, particularly assisted reproduction, is dependent on maternal age. The three main determining factors will be whether the woman is symptomatic from the endometriosis, the severity and distribution of the endometriosis and the coexistence of any other pathology contributing to subfertility. In an asymptomatic woman with mild endometriosis, laparoscopic treatment of the endometriosis may improve fertility. However, if the nature of the endometriosis is not amenable to surgery, the delay associated with medical treatment may not be justified. In women who are symptomatic or who have moderate to severe endometriosis, treatment of the endometriosis should take priority. Surgical management has the advantage over medical treatment of being completed quickly and giving longer-acting results. Ideally, this is best performed by laparoscopic laser or diathermy, as there is decreased patient morbidity and adhesion formation is less. Deroofing and cystectomy of an endometriotic ovarian cyst is possible laparoscopically, but an open procedure may be required. The surgical objective of removing endometriosis must be balanced against the need to conserve ovarian tissue for reproduction. In severe disease, medical treatment may be required in addition to surgery, to mop up residual disease. In mild to moderate endometriosis or when endometrial deposits are not suitable for surgery (for example, close proximity to a ureter), medical treatment may be chosen as a first-line treatment. Amenorrhoea must be maintained for at least 6 months and, in the majority, symptoms recur within 12 months of cessation. The combined oral contraceptive pill and continuous medroxyprogesterone acetate regimes are well tolerated, but they are less effective than danazol or GnRH (gonadotrophin releasing hormone) analogues. Danazol is often not tolerated, owing to androgenic side-effects. Despite climacteric side-effects, GnRH analogues are better tolerated and the risk of osteoporosis can be offset by the use of add-back hormone replacement therapy. Further laparoscopic assessment is required, following medical treatment, to assess outcome.

Comments
The question is obviously angled at your grasp of the current knowledge regarding the association between infertility and endometriosis.

Once again, treat this as a clinical problem and discuss your rationale in prioritising the management. After all, the question suggests that the woman is asymptomatic and her main concern is primary infertility.

This is still an infertility question. Remember to mention the partner.

The question omits the degree and extent of the disease. Obviously the other omissions are the results of the remaining infertility investigations, as these may also influence management.

Suggested reading
American Fertility Society 1985 Revised American Fertility Society classification of endometriosis. Fertility and Sterility 43: 351–352

Rock J A 1995 Endometriosis: critical developments in understanding and management. International Journal of Gynaecology and Obstetrics 50(suppl 1): 1–42

Shaw R W 1991 Treatment of endometriosis. In: Studd J (ed) Progress in obstetrics and gynaecology. Churchill Livingstone, Edinburgh, vol 9, pp 273–287

5. **A primiparous woman presents 2 months postnatally, complaining of persistent dyspareunia. Explore further management.**

Management depends on careful assessment by a full history and examination. Important details include whether this predates or dates from the delivery and whether this is superficial or deep dyspareunia. Enquiry must be made regarding associated symptoms such as vaginal discharge or bleeding and pelvic pain. It is essential to review the notes, obtaining as much information as possible about the delivery, whether she had an episiotomy or a tear and whether there was any difficulty in suturing and securing haemostasis. The experience of the operator and any postnatal complications are also relevant information.

Having obtained a full history, a gentle examination of the vulva and vagina is important, noticing any scar tissue or fibrosis resulting from a perineal repair. In particular, the capacity of the introitus, the presence of an unsupported skin bridge at the fourchette and the site of any discomfort is significant. A speculum examination may reveal granulation tissue (which can be cauterised) and a bimanual examination is important to assess pelvic pathology causing deep dyspareunia. If infection is suspected, high vaginal and endocervical culture swabs and an endocervical chlamydial swab should be taken. If the problem appears to be deep dyspareunia, a laparoscopy should be considered. If the cause is perineal scarring, the patient should be counselled and consent obtained for examination under general or regional anaesthesia and refashioning of the repair. If there is any scar tissue causing narrowing of the introitus, this should be removed, an interrupted polyglycolic acid suture performed and haemostasis ensured. Polyglycolic sutures excite less tissue reaction than those based on catgut. In some cases, a Fenton's procedure may be necessary, to deal with an unsupported skin bridge. Breastfeeding can cause some dryness of the vagina and vulva, due to high prolactin and low oestrogen, but this is usually later than 2 months postnatally. Vaginal dryness, in conjunction with the decreased libido often present at this time, can lead to significant dyspareunia. Careful counselling and reassurance is essential in this situation. In all cases, advice regarding lubrication prior to penetration during sexual intercourse is important.

Comments
Clinical points to be covered (that have been omitted from the question) include differentiation between deep and superficial dyspareunia, whether the dyspareunia predated the delivery, and details of the delivery and perineal repair.

Diagnostic laparoscopy to investigate deep dyspareunia is essential. Although it is likely that this case is related to an episiotomy scar following her delivery, other causes of dyspareunia should not be forgotten.

Suggested reading
Reader F 1991 Disorders of female sexuality. In: Studd J (ed) Progress in obstetrics and gynaecology. Churchill Livingstone, Edinburgh, vol 9, pp 303–317

PAPER 5

1. How can we avoid litigation in gynaecological surgery?

Litigation is an increasing problem in all branches of surgery and gynaecology is no exception. There are, however, many recognised ways of reducing the risk of successful litigation, preoperatively, intraoperatively and postoperatively. The introduction of a *clinical risk management system*, which may include critical event reporting and the appointment of a clinical risk officer, may reduce the incidence of litigation and has been widely introduced in the United States of America. The most important general points are careful *documentation* in the medical notes and effective *communication* with the patient. Preoperatively, it is important to build a rapport with patient and family and to ensure they have an accurate understanding of the nature and aims of an operation, as well as the possible complications. This must be documented fully. A patient information leaflet is helpful. Only after this can 'informed consent' be obtained. The surgeon should see each patient on admission, prior to premedication, to ensure the operation is still appropriate and consolidate previous counselling. Local protocols must be followed regarding patient identity checks, consent forms and the provision of results of preoperative investigations. Intraoperatively, the operating list must be supervised by an experienced surgeon. An appropriate grade of assistant should be available in accordance with General Medical Council guidelines. Recognition of complications, prompt action and early involvement of senior staff and multidisciplinary input when required are the key points in intraoperative care. A comprehensive operation note is essential, as is full postoperative counselling regarding the implications of any complication. Postoperatively, successful litigation often occurs as a result of delayed diagnosis and action (for example delayed diagnosis of ureteric injury). Development of protocols and clinical pathways and a good chain of communication from nursing and junior medical staff to senior surgeons can reduce this occurrence. In the case of day surgery, postoperative counselling is difficult as time is limited and the patient still recovering from the influence of anaesthesia. Therefore, a repeat discussion in the outpatient clinic may be required. Operative details should be provided via a prompt discharge letter to the general practitioner, including details of any investigations (particularly histology).

Comments

When approaching such a question, it is important to be able to break down your answer to give the impression of a methodical and therefore a comprehensive approach: in this example, preoperative, intraoperative and postoperative were chosen.

Now write an essay plan for the equivalent essay in obstetrics.

Suggested reading

Senior O E, Symonds E M 1995 Medical risk management: a prototype. Current Obstetrics and Gynaecology 5: 119–121

Stanhope N 1997 Applying human factors and methods to clinical risk management in obstetrics. British Journal of Obstetrics and Gynaecology 104: 1225–1232

2. Critically appraise the treatment options for a confirmed tubal pregnancy.

This has been an active area of recent development in the search to reduce the associated morbidity and the consequences for future fertility of this common gynaecological emergency. The options lie between surgical and non-surgical approaches. Surgery can be approached by the open or laparoscopic techniques and may involve salpingectomy or tubal conservation. Following resuscitation, conventional open salpingectomy is the accepted approach in cases of a ruptured tubal pregnancy, as rapid access and control of blood loss is the highest priority. Haemorrhage from ectopic pregnancy remains a significant cause of maternal mortality. Laparoscopic surgery is also unsuitable for a surgeon who is inexperienced laparoscopically, where appropriate equipment is unavailable or in the presence of an ectopic of greater than 5 cm in diameter, a cornual ectopic or dense adhesions. In suitable cases, the laparoscopic approach leads to decreased morbidity and early discharge and may be cosmetically superior. Conservative surgery aims to conserve the affected tube to aid future fertility. Partial salpingectomy is of value if the ectopic pregnancy is situated in the isthmic or ampullary region of the tube and if the other tube is damaged or absent. Anastomosis of the remnants of fallopian tube can be performed at the time or at a later date, allowing further conception. Further ectopic pregnancy can occur at the site of re-anastomosis or in a residual tubal remnant. Small intact isthmic or ampullary tubal pregnancies may be suitable for linear salpingostomy. There appears to be no advantage in closing the tube following salpingostomy. A pregnancy at the fimbrial end may be expressed. Direct injection of the ectopic pregnancy by hyperosmolar glucose, prostaglandin $F_{2\alpha}$ and methotrexate or intramuscular methotrexate have been used with varying success. Success is low with large ectopic pregnancies, 20% requiring surgery. All cases where the fallopian tube is conserved result in a high level of recurrent ectopic pregnancy (10%), but in addition, where the implantation site of the ectopic is conserved, there is a risk of residual trophoblastic tissue. All cases of conservative surgery of this type must be followed up with serial serum beta human chorionic gonadotrophin estimation.

Comments
The answer should be confined to treatment only. Make sure you don't waste time including details of diagnosis etc., particularly since this question also used the word 'confirmed'.

Application of information from the latest Confidential Enquiries into Maternal Death will be well received and may get you any discretionary points available.

Suggested reading
D'Mello M, Wingfield M 1997 Laparoscopic management of tubal ectopic pregnancies: the Irish experience. Irish Medical Journal 90: 182–183
Powell M P, Spellman J R 1996 Medical management of the patient with an ectopic pregnancy. Journal of Perinatal and Neonatal Nursing 9: 31–43

3. **What impact has the advent of evidence-based practice had on the management of menorrhagia?**

The idea behind evidence-based practice is that clinical management is determined by careful consideration of research evidence available, the most weight being given to randomised controlled trials.

Menorrhagia is a common and debilitating condition and there is no ideal treatment. There are concerns regarding the efficacy of medical treatment and the morbidity associated with surgical treatment. Many time-honoured diagnostic and therapeutic methods have only recently been adequately evaluated in research trials. The management of menorrhagia has been marked by the rapid and enthusiastic introduction of novel treatments without adequate prior research.

Research has questioned the use of the dilatation and curettage (D&C) in women under 45 years old. In the absence of intermenstrual or postcoital bleeding, pathology is rare. Even where further investigation is necessary, transvaginal ultrasound and outpatient endometrial sampling are being evaluated. Research has demonstrated the limitations of a D&C as a diagnostic tool. As it is a blind procedure, part of the cavity is often missed in the curettage and therefore accompanying hysteroscopy has been endorsed.

The traditional medical treatment of cyclical progesterone produces a predictable bleeding pattern, but quantitative assay demonstrates that it is ineffective in reducing menstrual loss. However, similar research demonstrates the effectiveness of tranexamic acid.

Reduction in menstrual loss has been proven objectively with the progesterone-releasing intrauterine device, a particularly suitable method in women requiring contraception. The long-term data regarding patient satisfaction following transcervical resection and laser ablation of the endometrium have been disappointing. New techniques also using endometrial destruction, such as thermal balloon therapy, should be introduced more circumspectly when the long-term data from randomised controlled trials are available. Minimal-access techniques such as laparoscopic hysterectomy and laparoscopically assisted vaginal hysterectomy (LAVH) initially achieved popularity. The hope was that these techniques would replace abdominal hysterectomy, achieving equally high patient satisfaction, but with lower morbidity and inpatient stay. However, re-evaluation of these techniques in comparison with vaginal hysterectomy has revealed that vaginal hysterectomy is quicker and achieves equally good results, without the use of expensive equipment.

Comments

This is an extremely topical subject. Make sure that you are aware of the principles of evidence-based practice.

The question stated management and therefore you must include examples from diagnostic methods as well as treatments.

Critical reading and evidence-based practice are likely new RCOG oral assessment examination stations.

4. A 36-year-old woman has dysfunctional uterine bleeding. She expresses a wish to avoid hysterectomy. Evaluate the range of treatment options available.

The choice of treatment lies between medical and other surgical options and must be tailored according to the individual case. Assessment should include the impact of her symptoms on her quality of life. Her concerns regarding hysterectomy need to be explored. There are several choices for medical treatment. Inhibitors of fibrinolysis (tranexamic acid) and prostaglandin synthetase inhibitors (mefenamic acid) are effective in reducing menstrual loss. As they are just taken at the time of menses, they do not interfere with conception. Ethamsylate is another option, acting by reducing capillary fragility, but it has not achieved popularity because it relies on assuming normal platelet function. Cyclical progesterone and the combined low-dose oral contraceptive pill (OCP), are well tolerated and produce good cycle control, but have less effect on menorrhagia. The OCP would be inadvisable if this woman is a smoker. The progesterone-releasing coil appears to be an exciting alternative in the treatment of menorrhagia, producing a reduction in the mean menstrual blood loss and the duration of menstruation. However, many are removed due to irregular bleeding, they are expensive and they are unsuitable for the nulliparous and those patients aiming for a pregnancy. Other medical options include danazol, which is poorly tolerated due to the androgenic side-effects, whereas the gonadotrophin releasing hormone agonists cause osteoporosis. Both are therefore unsuitable for long-term use. The surgical alternatives, though conserving the uterus, involve endometrial destruction and therefore should not be used if fertility is an issue. The common techniques used are transcervical resection of the endometrium and laser ablation. Radiofrequency ablation is hazardous except in experienced hands and thus has not achieved popularity. These operations avoid any scars and have reduced morbidity in comparison to hysterectomy, but around 15% of women are dissatisfied with the result. Long-term outcome is uncertain and there is a theoretical risk of late presentation of endometrial carcinoma due to concealed bleeding. If this woman also has dysmenorrhoea, conservative surgery is unlikely to be effective, owing to the possibility of adenomyosis. If this woman's main concern regarding hysterectomy is cosmetic, a vaginal hysterectomy may be considered.

Comments
The answer must be focused on treatment options only. No discussion should be entered into regarding uterine fibroids etc., as the diagnosis of dysfunctional uterine bleeding is stated specifically in the question.

The question obviously calls for a broad coverage of all alternatives (medical and surgical), not an in-depth view of any particular option. However, this must be treated as a clinical problem. The question omits the reasons behind this woman's wish to avoid hysterectomy. If there is a desire to preserve fertility, treatment is limited to medical treatment

Suggested reading
Lewis B V 1989 Hysteroscopy. In: Studd J (ed) Progress in obstetrics and gynaecology. Churchill Livingstone, Edinburgh, vol 7, pp 305–318

Mints M, Raderstad A, Rylander E 1998 Follow up of hysteroscopic surgery for menorrhagia. Acta Obstetrica et Gynecologica Scandinavica 77: 435–438

Pinion S B, Kitchener H C 1992 Conservative alternative to hysterectomy. Current Obstetrics and Gynaecology 2: 141–145

Sharp N C 1998 Endometrial ablation: future methods and novel treatments. Current Obstetrics and Gynaecology 8: 85–89

5. **An obese 34-year-old woman was referred by her general practitioner because of oligomenorrhoea and excessive hair growth. Outline further management.**

The pattern of oligomenorrhoea, hirsutism and obesity is classically and most commonly found in polycystic ovarian syndrome (PCOS), but may also be found in rarer disorders such as adrenal tumours. The woman's main concerns will determine management strategy. A full history and examination should be completed. The presence of acne, infertility or acanthosis nigricans (associated with insulin resistance) supports the diagnosis of PCOS. Symptoms and signs of overt virilism, such as temporal hair recession, clitoromegaly, voice changes, male body habitus and breast atrophy should raise suspicion of other pathology. Investigations should include thyroid function, prolactin, luteinising hormone (LH), follicle stimulating hormone (FSH), serum testosterone, androstenedione and pelvic ultrasound scan. Raised testosterone, androstenedione, LH and the polycystic appearance of the ovaries confirm PCOS. A glucose tolerance test and lipid profile should be considered, as abnormal lipids and maturity-onset diabetes is a significant risk. In significant virilism, and where the serum testosterone is greater than 5 nmol/L, Cushing's syndrome, late-onset adrenal hyperplasia or androgen-producing tumours of the adrenal or ovary must be excluded. Obesity has an influence on anovulation, hirsutism and the chance of developing diabetes. Weight reduction is therefore an important part of any treatment strategy of a woman with PCOS. In the long term, oligomenorrhoea is thought to be associated with an increased incidence of endometrial hyperplasia and carcinoma. Ensuring regular menses can reduce the risk, for example by the use of the combined oral contraceptive pill (where fertility is not an issue). Hirsutism or acne can be improved by a regime containing cyproterone acetate, such as the oral contraceptive Dianette or the reversed sequential regime which also induces regular menstruation. Spironolactone provides an alternative approach for those women whose hirsutism is unresponsive to cyproterone acetate. All these can be supplemented by hair removal, e.g. by electrolysis. In cases of subfertility or recurrent miscarriage, comprehensive investigation should be performed. Subfertility secondary to anovulation can be managed initially with an antioestrogen such as clomiphene citrate. Often PCOS is resistant to clomiphene and carefully monitored gonadotrophin induction of ovulation, ovarian diathermy or drilling, or assisted reproduction may be considered.

Comments
Although no diagnosis was stipulated, the answer should obviously concentrate on polycystic ovarian syndrome, as the other possibilities are rare.

Mentioning the aetiology etc. will not get points. Did you concentrate on management alone?

Note how polycystic ovarian syndrome must be written in full: 'polycystic ovarian syndrome (PCOS)' the first time it is mentioned. Thereafter, the abbreviation can be used.

A good exercise is to devise checklists of important management points for particular clinical presentations whilst in the gynaecology clinic.

Suggested reading

Eden J A 1989 The polycystic ovary syndrome. Australia and New Zealand Journal of Obstetrics and Gynaecology 29(4): 403–416

Franks S 1995 Polycystic ovary syndrome. New England Journal of Medicine 333: 853–861

PAPER 6

1. A 5-year-old girl presents with a 2-week history of offensive profuse vaginal discharge. Justify your management strategy.

Ideally, the girl should be seen with her mother and time allowed to build a rapport and gain the confidence of parent and child. The assessment must begin with a full history. In all cases of vaginal infection in a child, the possibility of sexual abuse should be remembered and therefore the clinician must remain alert for inconsistencies in the history and examination. In this age group, the vaginal resistance to infection has not fully developed. Details of the discharge should be taken, such as the colour, amount, duration and associated odour or itchiness. Examination in the outpatient setting should be restricted to a general examination and inspection of the external genitalia. Particular note should be made of any discharge from the introitus and if possible a sample should be sent for culture and sensitivity. Any excoriation or other trauma should be noted. If the dominant symptom is itching, the possibility of threadworms should not be forgotten. Diagnostic imaging such as ultrasound or X-ray is of use if a pelvic mass or a radio-opaque foreign body is suspected. Where the vaginal discharge is bloodstained or there is a history of a foreign object, further examination is indicated. Further examination must be performed under general anaesthesia by an experienced gynaecologist. Good visualisation of the vagina is difficult and the options lie between a head lamp and nasal speculum, a paediatric laryngoscope or the endoscopic approach, which is an increasingly popular option. A bimanual examination would be performed by the per rectal route. Once again, culture swabs must be taken from introitus and vagina. A foreign body must be removed and sent for culture itself. Rarely there can be tumours, such as embryonal rhabdomyosarcoma (sarcoma botryoides). Any suspected lesion must be biopsied. The prognosis of these tumours has improved recently. Sarcoma botryoides is sensitive to modern chemotherapeutic agents. If a bacterial infection is suspected, clinically wide-spectrum antibiotics are essential, adjusted according to sensitivities once the swab results are available. Antifungal therapy should include an oral agent in addition to topical treatment to decrease gut colonisation and therefore the chance of reinfection. It is important to arrange follow-up to check that the discharge has fully resolved.

Comments

If you feel at a loss as to how to start the question owing to lack of experience in this field, begin by breaking the question down into basics. History, examination, investigation, diagnosis, treatment.

The examiner is, of course, interested in your clinical management of the problem, but he will be looking for general points regarding the management of a 5-year-old child. Did you remember the points made in Paper 4, Question 2?

Always remember that common problems are common. Don't write a page on very rare tumours and omit infection or foreign bodies.

Suggested reading
This is a textbook question so reread the section in the gynaecology textbook you have chosen.

2. **Evaluate the place of the menorrhagia clinic in modern gynaecological practice.**

The workload currently posed by women suffering from menorrhagia is considerable, making up around 5% of consultations in general practice and 60% of gynaecological referrals. The current pattern of care is criticised as being inefficient, costly and time-consuming. A specialist menorrhagia clinic is considered to be a superior alternative.

This type of clinic is popular with general practitioners, as it allows a more streamlined approach to care and it empowers the general practitioner, permitting easier access to a diagnostic service and specialist opinion. A greater throughput of referrals can be achieved with fewer inpatient episodes and hospital visits, with attendant cost saving. Improved quality of care can be delivered by the additional input of trained nurse practitioners, allowing improved patient communication and an integrated care package. Careful audit of the management of menorrhagia is facilitated in this setting, allowing the audit of new measures and adjustment accordingly. However, the equipment required, such as an ultrasound machine (with transvaginal probe) and hysteroscopes, as well as suitable facilities, requires considerable capital cost. The training of suitable staff and the education of general practitioners is time-consuming and expensive but essential. Without the introduction of a suitable protocol and care pathway and the adherence of general practitioners to strict referral criteria, the workload can actually increase. This is due to inappropriate referrals and can even culminate in unnecessary procedures. A menorrhagia clinic is not able to deal with all patients and will always be dependent on the availability of traditional outpatient and inpatient facilities. Some patients will still require several visits to discuss their problem, whilst others will be unsuitable for outpatient procedures. Around 3–4% of outpatient hysteroscopies cannot be satisfactorily completed because of patient anxiety or for technical reasons.

Comments
It is important to write an essay plan because it is essential to answer this in a methodical way.

Think of other examples of this type of question (e.g. the day surgery unit) and write appropriate essay plans for practice.

If stuck for something to write about, remember issues such as training, reduction in hospital visits, cost-effectiveness, research and audit.

Suggested reading
Effective Health Care 1995 The management of menorrhagia. University of Leeds, Leeds
Tindall V R 1990 Jeffcoate's principles of gynaecology, 5th edn. Butterworths, London

3. **During ovulation induction, a 34-year-old woman becomes ill and collapses. How would you approach subsequent management?**

Resuscitation and the emergency management of this collapsed patient should initially take priority over other issues. Management must be headed by an experienced gynaecologist, with multidisciplinary input when appropriate. Oxygen should be given and the patient positioned appropriately (semi-erect in cardiorespiratory compromise, or supine in hypovolaemic shock). A blood glucose and 12-lead electrocardiogram should be performed and arterial blood gases and pulse oximetry considered as an emergency. Blood samples should be taken for a full blood count, urea, creatinine, electrolytes, clotting and a group and save, and intravenous access established. Although the complications arising from severe ovarian hyperstimulation syndrome (OHSS) is the most likely diagnosis, the time scale may suggest a pregnancy-related complication. Coincidental pathology must not be left out of the differential diagnosis (for example, diabetic ketoacidosis). There is a significant risk of a ruptured or bleeding ovarian cyst, respiratory decompensation due to splinting of the diaphragm and pleural effusions, thromboembolic stroke or pulmonary embolism in OHSS. A history should be taken from patient or partner. Hyperstimulation is more likely in a woman with polycystic ovarian syndrome, a history of OHSS, during an in vitro fertilisation supraovulation cycle (high risk if there are a large number of harvested follicles, high oestradiol levels and if embryo transfer performed) and with human chorionic gonadotrophin (hCG) support. Notably, it is also associated with successful conception, which must be borne in mind during further management. On examination, signs of OHSS include ascites, pleural and pericardial effusions and dehydration. These are confirmed on chest X-ray and ultrasound examination. Serum albumin is low and the haematocrit and urea high. The basic principles of management of severe OHSS include appropriate analgesia, careful fluid balance, thromboembolic prophylaxis with stockings and subcutaneous heparin. Fluid replacement should be colloid or albumin infusion and may require central venous pressure monitoring. Diuretics must be avoided as they cause further haemoconcentration. In respiratory compromise, a therapeutic paracentesis or drainage of pleural effusions may be required. hCG support should be converted to progesterone. If OHSS fails to resolve and a pregnancy is ongoing, termination may rarely be required.

Comments
Demonstrate your ability to prioritise: emergency priorities first.

Yes! It does initially seem like a subspeciality question, but any district general hospital must be competent in the management of this condition, as the patient may be many miles from her treatment centre.

'Safe doctor' points. All collapsed patients should have a blood glucose estimate performed. Diuretics will cause increased intravascular dehydration and the increased viscosity and hypercoagulability can precipitate thromboembolism.

Suggested reading
Balasch J 1996 Treatment of severe ovarian hyperstimulation syndrome by a conservative medical approach. Acta Obstetrica et Gynecologica Scandinavica 75: 662–667
McClure N, Healy D L 1991 Ovarian hyperstimulation syndrome. Lancet 338: 1111–1112

4. A 25-year-old woman presents requesting sterilisation. Discuss her preoperative management and counselling.

This is not an uncommon request in women of this age, despite the wide range of contraceptive choices available. A detailed history should be taken and, in particular, the reasons behind the request should be fully explored. Parity, past obstetric history, social circumstances, difficulty with other forms of contraception and the presence of a stable relationship may all lend support to the case for performing sterilisation. This should be followed by a full examination (including a speculum and bimanual examination) to exclude any coexistent pathology that may complicate the procedure. Careful counselling is mandatory in any woman considering sterilisation and preferably should also involve her partner. The most important point (particularly in a 25-year-old woman) is that sterilisation must be considered as irreversible. Alternatives such as vasectomy of her partner and reversible methods, including the progesterone-releasing implant and intrauterine device (which have comparable contraceptive success to sterilisation) should be discussed. Although both male and female sterilisation have a low morbidity, female sterilisation carries a higher risk, as the procedure is intra-abdominal and cannot be performed under a local anaesthetic. The risk of failure of the procedure of 1–2 per 1000 must be emphasised (1 per 200 if performed at the time of caesarean section). The woman must be warned to present early for medical attention should she have a positive pregnancy test, as the incidence of ectopic pregnancy is higher following failed sterilisation. The nature of the procedure should be explained. In the majority of cases, the laparoscopic method will be the aim. All women should be warned of the possibility of conversion of the procedure to a mini-laparotomy in cases of unforeseen difficulties, but in the very obese or those with adhesions, 'minilap' sterilisation is the method of first choice. Menstrual sequelae (usually as a consequence of cessation of hormonal contraception rather than a direct consequence of the procedure) should be covered. All this information must be reiterated on admission, prior to premedication, and informed consent (using specific consent forms for sterilisation) obtained. Documentation of counselling must be clearly recorded, as this is one of the most common areas for claims for medical litigation.

Comments
This is a very basic question, so the standard required will be high. We know little about this woman. Is she parous? What is her obstetric history? Does she have health problems? Has she tried other forms of contraception? Is she fat? Has she had previous surgery? Remember the partner.

The age has obviously been chosen to introduce controversy. The irreversible nature of the procedure is obviously of concern in a young woman.

This would also be suitable as a counselling station in the new RCOG oral assessment examination, as would a woman requesting IUCD, OCP, etc. Make checklists of the points you would include. Practice these orally prior to the OSCE.

Suggested reading
Filshie G M 1995 Update in female sterilisation. Current Obstetrics and Gynaecology 5: 169–173

5. **A 60-year-old widow presents with recurrent offensive vaginal discharge. Discuss the further management of this case.**

Assessment of this case must start with the taking of a full history and performing a full examination. The most common cause is that of atrophic vaginitis, infection of the vagina due to susceptibility of the vagina secondary to low oestrogen. Benign pathology, such as cervical or endometrial polyps, can also present with a discharge. However, malignancy of the cervix, endometrium and rarely the fallopian tube can present this way. Senile endometritis can occur as a result of senile vaginitis or secondary to endometrial cancer and can culminate in pyometra. Rectovaginal fistulae present with a very offensive discharge and are usually secondary to bowel malignancy or previous radiotherapy, though they can be secondary to genital tract malignancy. A detailed history of the discharge should be obtained, in particular regarding the colour, amount, duration, associated odour and itchiness. The history should also include associated symptoms, past gynaecological problems, smear history, menopausal and hormone replacement therapy details, obstetric history and a review of urinary and gastrointestinal symptoms. A history of previous radiotherapy is extremely important. An important aspect is to sensitively enquire regarding the woman's current sexual relationships, as a new relationship can still result in a sexually transmitted infection, despite the older age group. Examination should include abdominal, speculum and bimanual examination. A high vaginal swab, endocervical swab and cervical smear should be taken. An ultrasound scan examination can be used to investigate a pelvic mass and to measure endometrial thickness (an irregular or endometrial thickness of greater than 5 mm being indicative of pathology). The investigative gold standard is hysteroscopy and endometrial biopsy. Treatment depends on the underlying pathology. Once malignancy has been excluded, atrophic vaginitis can be treated with oestrogens, usually topically. A sexually transmitted infection requires referral to the genitourinary clinic for contact tracing and a full screening. A pyometra is usually resolved by a dilatation and curettage. Should it recur, however, a hysterectomy may be indicated, as there may be an occult endometrial carcinoma. Polyps can be removed at the time of hysteroscopy.

Comments
A textbook question testing your basic gynaecology skills. To score highly, a systematic logical approach encompassing all possible

diagnoses is essential. It is useful to mentally classify the causes anatomically: vaginal, cervical, uterine, etc. first so that you don't miss any possibility.

'Safe doctor' point. Avoid the use of oestrogens until endometrial carcinoma has been excluded.

Suggested reading
This is a textbook question, so reread the section in the gynaecology textbook you have chosen.

PAPER 7

1. Debate the impact of the early pregnancy assessment unit.

The aim of the early pregnancy unit was to improve quality of patient care in an atmosphere of scarce resources. In this context, the early pregnancy unit has the ability to make a considerable positive impact. In the past, the most junior doctor would admit emergencies, initiate investigations and treatment and the patient would have to await senior review before any further step could be taken. Reliance on emergency operating time and the low priority placed on miscarriage cases in comparison to life-threatening cases often culminated in a stressful, costly and prolonged period in hospital. The aim of an early pregnancy assessment unit is to provide a well-equipped service to deal with early pregnancy problems, avoiding such a waste of resources. The unit being open during the day, throughout the week (i.e. 7 days) accomplishes this. The unit must be adequately staffed by experienced nursing staff, and senior gynaecological cover must be available for the junior medical staff involved. There must be strict protocols in place for referral criteria and management. Rapid access to ultrasound scan examination, pregnancy testing and haematological services is essential, to allow rapid throughput. The unit should be a dedicated suite, with privacy available for counselling. This type of unit can deal with a range of gynaecological problems effectively, including miscarriage and ectopic pregnancy. There is early access to counselling and viability scanning, with reassurance for patients with previous ectopic pregnancy and recurrent miscarriage. The scope can even be broadened to providing streamlined care for other acute gynaecological conditions, such as Bartholin's cysts and abscesses. The centralisation of services allows data collection and facilitates research. However, unless this service is carefully planned, there can be a negative effect. The capital cost is high and benefits may not be realised unless strict protocols are adhered to. If casualty and primary care services are not involved in planning, there may be an increase in unnecessary referral, as such a service may lower their threshold for referral. Unless an audit process is in place at the beginning, the service will not be responsive to the changing needs of the population served.

Comments

This is the latest thinking in acute gynaecology. As such, there has been quite a bit of discussion in the medical news. If this has managed to pass you by, just think carefully of what advantages this would have for the patient and the hospital and then the potential disadvantages. If you find the question difficult, remember there will be others who find the question impossible, so make an attempt.

When you have finished your list of clinical pros and cons, don't forget points such as cost-effectiveness, research and audit.

Suggested reading

Draycott T J, Read M D 1996 The role of early pregnancy assessment clinics. Current Obstetrics and Gynaecology 6: 148–152

2. A 74-year-old woman has confirmed advanced ovarian carcinoma. How would you approach her care?

Ovarian carcinoma is often silent and rapidly progressive and as there is no effective screening test, initial presentation with advanced disease is unfortunately not uncommon. The discussion with patient and family must be open, but conducted at the patient's pace. Counselling must be provided by an experienced counsellor. The opinion of the gynae-oncologist should be sought as, on occasions, palliative chemotherapy may be considered, though debulking surgery and therapeutic chemotherapy are unlikely to be considered. Care should largely be determined by symptom relief. Adequate pain relief is important and should be initiated and increased in accordance with an analgesia ladder until the patient is pain-free. In this, simple analgesics such as regular paracetamol or non-steroidal anti-inflammatory drugs occupy the bottom rung, morphine the middle rung and diamorphine the top rung. In cases of troublesome vomiting, the rectal, transdermal, subcutaneous or parenteral route can be used. If there are difficulties experienced in obtaining satisfactory pain control, the advice of the pain control clinic should be sought. An anti-emetic can be used, such as prochlorperazine. The effective ondansetron ($5HT_3$ antagonist) may be used. However, in intractable vomiting, an intravenous infusion will need to be started and electrolyte correction performed. Attention as to the cause is important, as bowel obstruction is not unlikely. Following careful counselling, a palliative colostomy may be performed. The symptom relief must be carefully balanced against the operation morbidity. Constipation is a common problem, particularly with opiate administration, and should be pre-empted by regular laxative administration. Abdominal discomfort and dyspnoea is common, secondary to ascites, and palliative paracentesis is often indicated. Early involvement of the primary care team and the Macmillan nurses is essential as, prior to leaving the ward, there should be watertight arrangements for the family to gain rapid assistance in case of deterioration. If the family are ready to make decisions regarding the place of terminal care, then preliminary arrangements can be made, such as referral for a hospice place. In addition, there should be follow-up arrangements in place, so that care can be continually monitored and modified.

Comments
Palliative care is as important as curative care and you must not forget this during your examination preparation. Although the trend is for treatment of ovarian cancer to be undertaken in major centres, palliative care obviously needs to be based locally and therefore all gynaecologists need a sound knowledge of palliative care.

   Note that the question makes the point of saying that this is *confirmed* advanced ovarian carcinoma and therefore it is steering you away from discussing staging, laparotomies, etc.

Suggested reading
British National Formulary 1998 Prescribing in palliative care. British Medical Association and Royal Pharmaceutical Society of Great Britain, London, September, pp 11–14

Burghardt (ed) 1993 Surgical gynaecological oncology. Thieme Medical
  Publications, Stuttgart
Coppleson M 1992 Gynaecological oncology, 2nd edn. Churchill
  Livingstone, Edinburgh

3. **A 17-year-old girl presents 14 hours after unprotected intercourse,
   requesting help. How would you proceed to manage this problem?**
   This is an important opportunity for intervention to modify this risk-taking
   behaviour. The establishment of a doctor–patient relationship in which
   she feels that her concerns will be treated with sympathy and in
   confidence is essential. A history should be taken, including details
   regarding previous contraceptive history, previous pregnancies and the
   last menstrual period. If there is a possibility of pregnancy conceived at
   an earlier date, this must be excluded before emergency contraception
   can be considered. The options for emergency contraception include
   either a hormonal method or the insertion of an intrauterine
   contraceptive device (IUCD). The well-established Yuzpe regime
   involves the oral administration of 100 µg ethinyl oestradiol and 0.5 mg
   levonorgestrel twice, 12 hours apart. The mode of action is uncertain,
   but it may prevent ovulation and/or prevent implantation. This method
   carries a failure rate of up to 7% and the associated side-effects are
   nausea in up to 50%, vomiting in 20%, breast tenderness, menorrhagia
   and headache. Absolute contraindications include a history of
   thrombosis or focal migraine at the time of presentation. The woman
   should be asked to return if she vomits the tablets, as replacement
   tablets can be given with an anti-emetic. Mifepristone (600 mg within
   72 hours) has been advocated as an alternative to the Yuzpe regime,
   with a good success rate and a lower incidence of side-effects. The
   alternative is the IUCD, which can be inserted up to 5 days after
   intercourse and has the advantage of catering for future contraceptive
   needs. This method is more effective than the hormonal one, with a
   failure rate of less than 1%, but it is unsuitable for nulliparous women.
   There are the established complications of IUCD insertion of pain and
   bleeding, perforation of the uterus, expulsion, infection, vaginal
   discharge and menorrhagia. A full discussion is required to discuss
   long-term contraception, and additional barrier contraception should be
   advocated to protect against sexually transmitted infection. The girl
   should be warned to return if her period is late or heavy, or if she
   experiences abdominal pain, lest the emergency contraception has
   failed.

Comments
It is important to cover not only the options for emergency
contraception, but also to mention future contraception and the use of
barrier contraception to protect against sexually transmitted disease.
  Look critically at the question. Parity has been omitted and therefore,
despite the young age, an IUCD may be a possibility.

Suggested reading
Glasier A, Thong K J, Dewar M et al 1992 Randomised trial of
  mifepristone (RU486) and high dose oestrogen–progestogen as an

emergency contraceptive. New England Journal of Medicine 327: 1041–1044

Glasier A 1993 Post coital contraception. Current Obstetrics and Gynaecology 3: 91–96

4. Review the treatment options available for premenstrual syndrome.

There are many therapies used for premenstrual syndrome, reflecting the difficulty experienced in finding an effective treatment. This is partially due to the unknown aetiology, but in addition, the symptoms of premenstrual syndrome are difficult to assess, there is often an overlay of depressive symptoms and the placebo effect of any treatment is high in this condition. The latter point supports the validity of a non-pharmacological approach to treatment in the first instance. A sympathetic approach, coupled with general advice regarding diet and lifestyle, may well be of benefit. A reduction in dietary fat has been shown to decrease cyclical mastalgia, as has evening primrose oil. Vitamin B_6 has been used extensively in premenstrual syndrome, but this is not evidence-based practice and there have been recent concerns regarding safety. Where the dominant symptom is that of mood disturbance, treatment with antidepressants may be worthwhile. First, there may be a background of depression. In addition, recent work has suggested that premenstrual syndrome is due to a deficiency of central serotonergic activity. A selective serotonin reuptake inhibitor should therefore be the antidepressant of choice. On the basis that inhibition or modulation of cyclical ovarian activity causes relief of premenstrual syndrome, cyclical progesterone alone, the combined oral contraceptive pill and oestrogen implants with cyclical progesterone (sometimes in conjunction with a testosterone implant) have had a good response in a limited number of women. Danazol has been used in cases of refractory cyclical mastalgia, but is often poorly tolerated. In cases of severe premenstrual syndrome, where other treatments have failed, suppression of the menstrual cycle by induction of an artificial menopause with gonadotrophin releasing hormone analogues can be effective. Side-effects can be minimised by the use of add-back hormone replacement therapy, but nevertheless the incidence of osteoporosis and the expense of this treatment limits its long-term usage. Should this be successful, however, this would endorse the induction of a surgical menopause by oophorectomy (usually with hysterectomy), followed by oestrogen replacement, particularly in older women in whom fertility is not an issue.

Comments

This is a difficult subject, as ideal management is far from clear. The question specifies premenstrual syndrome, a broader remit than premenstrual tension. However, it is focused on *current treatment options* only. Did you waste time including other management aspects?

'Review' is an unusual format for a short essay question, as it requires a broad review. To handle this type of question, avoid any in-depth analysis of a particular treatment option, but aim for a comprehensive coverage of all the possible options.

Suggested reading
Freeman E W 1996 Sertraline versus desipramine in the treatment of premenstrual syndrome: an open-label trial. Journal of Clinical Psychiatry 57: 7–11
Ozeren S 1997 Fluoxetine in the treatment of premenstrual syndrome. European Journal of Obstetrics, Gynaecology and Reproductive Biology 73: 167–170

5. **Following a total abdominal hysterectomy and bilateral salpingo-oophorectomy, a 49-year-old woman presents with vaginal vault prolapse. Explore further management.**

Vaginal vault prolapse can be a difficult and challenging problem. A history should include details regarding symptomatology, quality of life, sexual history, hormone replacement therapy and urinary and bowel symptoms. Occupational, social and smoking history are important. On examination, a mass or ascites (which predispose to prolapse) should be excluded and coexistent cystocoele or rectocoele documented. Advice should be given to reduce her risk of worsening prolapse, including weight reduction, stopping smoking, avoiding constipation and avoiding repetitive heavy lifting. Adequate oestrogen replacement must be given. Pelvic floor exercises are of limited use in vault prolapse, but may help any coexistent cystocoele or rectocoele. A woman who has minimal symptoms or is medically unfit may require no further action. The next non-surgical option involves the use of ring or shelf pessaries. Ring pessaries have the advantage of being easier to insert and remove and are less likely to produce ulceration, but a shelf pessary may produce better control, particularly in perineal deficiency. This relatively young woman is likely to be medically fit for surgery and sexually active. If she has significant symptoms, she will opt for operative repair. The traditional colporrhaphy will not be effective in correcting a vault prolapse and may cause unacceptable narrowing of the vagina, making coitus impossible. Sacral colpopexy is an effective operation (over 90% success) which can be performed by an open or laparoscopic approach. Mesh or fascia is used to fix the vaginal vault to the sacral promontory. The disadvantages are that the open procedure has a significant morbidity, the mesh can get infected and associated prolapse requires a separate vaginal procedure. Transvaginal sacrospinous colpopexy involves the vault being fixed to the sacrospinous ligament transvaginally. This is technically demanding and requires an experienced vaginal surgeon. The success rate is also over 90%, but it avoids the morbidity of an abdominal incision. Joint abdomino-perineal procedures have not achieved popularity, as they are not felt to have an advantage over other operative procedures. Colpocleisis and colpectomy are usually kept as a last resort and are likely to be unsuitable, as they do not preserve sexual function.

Comments
Be careful about the wording: the question is not restricted to surgical management.
Remember to discuss sexual function, particularly if operative repair is to be considered.

General principles regarding reduction of risk factors are important to improve the outlook postoperatively.

Suggested reading

Carey M P, Slack M C 1994 Vaginal vault prolapse following hysterectomy. In: Studd J (ed) Progress in obstetrics and gynaecology. Churchill Livingstone, Edinburgh, vol 11, pp 387–397

Schotri M S 1997 How to do it in surgery: laparoscopic sacral colpopexy. British Journal of Hospital Medicine 57: 514

PAPER 8

1. **A 38-year-old woman presents, worried about the chances of developing ovarian carcinoma. Her mother, and more recently her sister, have died of ovarian carcinoma in their 40s. How would you counsel her?**

The woman is likely to be anxious, therefore adequate, uninterrupted time must be allotted to explore all the patient's concerns fully. The occurrence of two cases of premenopausal advanced ovarian cancer in first-degree relatives is highly suggestive of a familial predisposition. A family history, including other related cancers (breast, colon or endometrium), bilateral tumours or multiple primary tumours, would lend weight to the possibility of a genetic predisposition to cancer. The regional genetics service may be able to provide genetic screening if the exact mutation has been identified in her relatives. Based on the family history alone, the woman may be given an estimated risk increased from 1 in 70 to 1 in 40. The options lie between hysterectomy and bilateral oophorectomy or surveillance. If the woman has not completed her family, or if she is medically unfit or averse to surgery, screening may be attempted. Current screening is unsatisfactory, as there is no premalignant disease in ovarian carcinoma and its aggressive nature means that the disease may progress to advanced disease between screening visits. The simplest screening involves regular pelvic examination to detect adnexal masses, but it is unlikely to pick up early disease. CA 125 is the most useful serum marker, as it is raised in over 80% of patients with ovarian cancer, but it is not specific (e.g. raised in endometriosis) and only 50% are raised in stage I disease. Vaginal ultrasound examination and colour flow imaging have the potential to pick up early disease and even to differentiate between benign and malignant conditions, but are expensive. A combination of these screening methods may be more useful than a single method. Prophylactic oophorectomy reduces the risk of ovarian carcinoma dramatically. This must be balanced against the operative risk, sterility, surgical menopause and residual risk of peritoneal adenocarcinoma. The effect of long-term oestrogen replacement on an individual with a potential predisposition to breast cancer is unknown, but the new selective oestrogen receptor modulator drugs may avoid this potential risk. The operative morbidity can be reduced by performing a laparoscopically assisted vaginal hysterectomy and bilateral oophorectomy.

Comments
You must be familiar with the screening methods for ovarian cancer and be able to discuss the pros and cons of each method.

This is not an uncommon presentation in a gynaecology clinic. Remember that a 1 in 40 risk may be considered to be low by some, but it is unlikely to be by the patient!

Another related topic is the role of routine prophylactic oophorectomy at the time of hysterectomy. Write an essay plan as an examination preparation exercise.

Suggested reading
Eccles D M 1996 The genetics of gynaecological malignancy. British
    Journal of Hospital Medicine 56(8): 416–419
Pilling D W 1997 Ovarian ultrasound. British Journal of Hospital
    Medicine 57(1/2): 15–18
Prys A, Oram D 1991 Screening for ovarian cancer. In: Studd J (ed)
    Progress in obstetrics and gynaecology. Churchill Livingstone,
    Edinburgh, vol 9, pp 349–373

2. **A 19-year-old woman presents requesting oral contraception.
She has insulin-dependent diabetes mellitus, but is well controlled.
Can you justify giving it to her?**

The combined oral contraceptive pill is a well-established, safe
preparation which produces good cycle control and has a low failure rate.
In the teenage population, it is an ideal choice, in that it requires no
conscious act at the time of coitus and this age group is prone to
risk-taking behaviour. There are advantages of taking the oral
contraceptive pill, such as a reduction of menorrhagia, dysmenorrhoea,
premenstrual tension, benign breast disease, pelvic inflammatory
disease and it also confers protection against ovarian and endometrial
malignancy. In this girl, careful consideration must be given to her insulin-
dependent diabetes mellitus. It will be essential to counsel appropriately
regarding the risk of the oral contraceptive pill on diabetes. The main
concern is that of the long-term risk of arterial disease. The presence of
additional risk factors would result in an unacceptably high risk.
Therefore, if this woman is a smoker, hypertensive, obese, or has a
strong family history of arterial disease, the oral contraceptive pill could
not be justified. In addition, the presence of diabetic nephropathy or
retinopathy (indicators of previous poor diabetic control) preclude its use,
as the oral contraceptive pill may cause worsening control. Counselling
should involve her partner. It is appropriate to discuss the alternatives
available, such as depot progesterone, the progesterone-only pill,
progesterone implants and, in the parous, the copper or progesterone-
releasing intrauterine contraceptive device. All these methods are well
established in insulin-dependent diabetes and are effective
contraceptives. Barrier contraception is also an alternative and should be
advocated as protection against sexually transmitted infections. All these
alternatives have their drawbacks and it may be that, following careful
counselling, the combined oral contraceptive remains the patient's first
choice. In the absence of the contraindications mentioned earlier, the oral
contraceptive pill (preferably 20 μg of ethinyl oestradiol) can then be
justified. The main aim, after all, is to prevent an unplanned pregnancy: a
serious risk for the patient in terms of diabetic control and complications
and for pregnancy outcome. Preconceptual preparation is of paramount
importance for a diabetic woman. Advice against smoking is essential.

Comments
The concept of risk/benefit assessment is central to this question. You
need to show that you appreciate that the risks posed by the various
contraceptive alternatives are low in comparison to that of an unplanned
pregnancy.

With any contraception question, it is important to give a clear account of all the alternatives available.

Remember about the prevention of sexually transmitted diseases by the use of the sheath.

Suggested reading

Tayob Y, Guillebaud J 1990 Barrier methods of contraception. In: Studd J (ed) Progress in obstetrics and gynaecology. Churchill Livingstone, Edinburgh, vol 8, pp 371–390

3. **Evaluate the role of vaginal hysterectomy in modern gynaecological practice.**

Vaginal hysterectomy accounts for one-third of all hysterectomies performed for non-malignant conditions in the United Kingdom. This traditional technique has recently enjoyed an increase in popularity, following the realisation that an experienced vaginal surgeon can achieve a similar low level of patient morbidity by vaginal hysterectomy as that of a laparoscopic hysterectomy, but in reduced operative time. The main use of vaginal hysterectomy remains when hysterectomy is required during prolapse surgery. Uterine prolapse is, however, the result of genital prolapse and not the cause, therefore other procedures in which the uterus is conserved, such as the Manchester repair, may be equally effective. The presence of uterine descent is not a prerequisite for vaginal hysterectomy in experienced hands. Realisation of this has led to its use being extended to hysterectomy for benign pathology, such as dysfunctional uterine bleeding. Vaginal hysterectomy has advantages over abdominal hysterectomy as it avoids an abdominal wound, is associated with lower morbidity, shorter hospital stay and improved cost-effectiveness. Vaginal hysterectomy is superior in some specific instances, such as vaginal intraepithelial neoplasia (VAIN), as the iodine-deficient area can be removed under direct vision. There are some recognised limitations to the vaginal hysterectomy, such as specific training, limited access such as a narrow subpubic arch, known adhesions (due to endometriosis, multiple abdominal operations or severe pelvic infection), etc., because of the increased operative difficulty by the vaginal route. Although the vaginal route has been used for malignancy, it is not the approved approach, as surgical staging (such as that required for endometrial carcinoma) is not possible. Some traditional contraindications to vaginal hysterectomy are being challenged. If difficulties are anticipated regarding oophorectomy by the vaginal route, laparoscopic assistance can be employed. The current evidence is that the abdominal route confers no advantage over the vaginal route in women with a history of previous caesarean section. Increased uterine size has always been a concern, but the advent of gonadotrophin releasing hormone analogues (GnRH agonists) to reduce fibroid size, and techniques such as bisection and morcellation have also permitted more vaginal hysterectomies.

Comments

Essentially this question means assessing the value of vaginal hysterectomy relative to other procedures, including abdominal hysterectomy, laparoscopic hysterectomy and conservative surgery such as endometrial resection or ablation. Headings which may be considered include the current importance or prevalence, the current usage, the current limitations and the potential role in the future.

The question is restricted to the 'role of' vaginal hysterectomy, so don't get carried away with operative details etc.

Suggested reading
Sheth S 1993 Vaginal hysterectomy. In: Studd J (ed) Progress in obstetrics and gynaecology. Churchill Livingstone, Edinburgh, vol 10, pp 317–340

4. **A 30-year-old woman has persistent pelvic pain and dyspareunia. A diagnostic laparoscopy reveals extensive active endometriosis, including involvement of the left ovary. Evaluate the treatment options.**

The treatment options depend on symptom severity, degree of ovarian involvement and her future plans for fertility. Treatment can be medical, surgical, or a combination of both. In minimal ovarian involvement, medical treatment may be selected as first-line treatment. Medical treatment is based on producing prolonged amenorrhoea, utilising the continuous oral contraceptive pill, progestogens, gestrinone, danazol or gonadotrophin releasing hormone analogues (GnRH-a). GnRH-a is the most effective agent and therefore appropriate for severe endometriosis. Add-back hormone replacement therapy (HRT) will minimise adverse effects without decreasing effectiveness. Laparoscopic surgery is becoming a common first-line therapy and surgery is indicated anyway, if there is significant ovarian involvement. Adhesiolysis, laser or diathermy ablation of endometriotic deposits and deroofing or cystectomy of an endometriotic ovarian cyst are producing good results with low patient morbidity and adhesion formation, in comparison to the open approach. Postoperative GnRH-a would be advisable to mop up residual disease. The recurrence in ovarian endometrioma is still high, therefore in these cases an oophorectomy is often required. The need for surgical treatment must be balanced against the need to conserve ovarian tissue for reproduction. Unilateral oophorectomy is sometimes the only answer, even in women with subfertility. Pain control, such as division of the uterosacral ligaments and presacral neurectomy, have been employed with varying success. As endometriosis usually recurs within the year, subfertility treatment should not be delayed following treatment cessation. Successful pregnancy would achieve significant further regression of endometriosis.

Some women, particularly those women who have completed their family, may opt for definitive surgery: total abdominal hysterectomy and bilateral oophorectomy. If the right ovary is macroscopically unaffected, it can be conserved, but the woman should be counselled regarding the possibility of recurrence, as there may be microscopic deposits. As the risk of bowel or ureteric damage is high in surgery for endometriosis, it must be performed by an experienced gynaecological surgeon, with general surgical or urological input as required. The chance of reactivation of endometriosis after total abdominal hysterectomy and bilateral salpingo-oophorectomy is low and therefore withholding HRT is not justified, particularly in a 30-year-old woman.

Comments

The omissions in the question include the woman's wishes regarding fertility and her parity.

The concept of ovarian endometriosis being resistant to treatment must be covered, particularly as the question specifically mentions ovarian involvement.

Although surgery is the likely primary treatment, the question asks for an evaluation of all options.

Suggested reading

Brosens I (ed) 1993 Endometriosis. Clinical Obstetrics and
  Gynaecology 7: 673–868
Shaw R W 1991 Treatment of endometriosis. In: Studd J (ed) Progress
  in obstetrics and gynaecology. Churchill Livingstone, Edinburgh,
  vol 9, pp 273–287

5. **A girl of 7 years presents with full development of secondary
   female sexual characteristics. Discuss further management.**

Precocious thelarche and pubarche is a difficult problem for both child and family, so a sympathetic and reassuring approach is essential. History should include enquiry regarding onset of menstruation, familial history, developmental history and past and current illness. In particular, a history of meningitis, encephalitis, a cerebral tumour or Albright's syndrome would be significant. Rarely, a careful history may reveal inadvertent exogenous oestrogen from medication or a dietary source.

Clinical examination must include a full general, as well as abdominal, examination and external inspection of the genitalia. Skeletal abnormalities and café au lait spots on the skin with Coast of Maine appearance are tell-tale features of Albright's disease. Investigations would include serum gonadotrophin levels, radiological investigation of the skull and abdomen and subsequent investigations as indicated.

Constitutional precocious puberty is the commonest cause and is due to premature release of gonadotrophins from the anterior pituitary. The exclusion of other pathology and high levels of gonadotrophins and oestradiol would suggest this. Premature release of gonadotrophins from the anterior pituitary may be due to a pathological process such as meningitis or encephalitis, or a cerebral tumour stimulating output. Computerised tomography of the head is useful. A skeletal survey is important if Albright's syndrome is suspected, as it is associated with polyostotic fibrous dysplasia. Overgrowth of the base of the skull accounts for the stimulation of the pituitary. A pelvic ultrasound scan may reveal a feminising tumour of the ovary (e.g. granulosa cell tumour). This would also be suggested by low levels of gonadotrophins with high oestrogen levels. In continued uncertainty, performance of a laparoscopy may be appropriate prior to laparotomy and tumour removal. The possibility of a follicular cyst secondary to constitutional puberty must be remembered. Adrenal cortical tumours and androgenic tumours of the ovary produce precocious virilism.

In all cases of development of secondary sexual characteristics, the parents must be warned of the increased risk of early sexual contact and associated pregnancy. Medroxyprogesterone acetate and danazol have been used to suppress menstruation and breast development. Cyprosterone acetate is the treatment of choice in Albright's disease. However, gonadotrophin releasing hormone analogues are the most effective treatment where inappropriate gonadotrophin release is the underlying cause.

Comments
Examination questions on paediatric gynaecology always cause consternation! Your examination preparation should include likely topics such as precocious/delayed puberty or menarche, vaginal discharge, genital injuries, sexual abuse and intersex conditions.

In this particular case, the question gives the examination findings and therefore description of how to perform a paediatric examination is unlikely to gain points.

Suggested reading
Lee P A 1994 Advances in the management of precocious puberty. Clinical Paediatrics 33: 54–61

Lincoln E A, Zuber T J 1998 Management of precocious puberty. Hospital Practitioner 33: 173–176

Wheeler M D, Styne D M 1990 Diagnosis and management of precocious puberty. Paediatric Clinical of North America 37: 1255–1271

PAPER 9

1. **A 59-year-old woman was referred by her general practitioner, who noticed a marked cystourethrocoele when taking a routine cervical smear. Justify your further management.**

The presence of a marked cystourethrocoele in this lady may or may not require treatment, depending on whether there were symptoms at the time of referral. Details must be taken of previous prolapse surgery, menopausal symptoms, urinary symptoms (such as incontinence, hesitancy, urgency, frequency and nocturia) and bowel symptoms (such as constipation). Past obstetric history may reveal difficult or prolonged deliveries. Intercurrent chest disease and smoking are significant risk factors. On examination, it is important to perform a general, as well as a local, examination. Prolapse can be secondary to intra-abdominal pathology. Vaginal examination should include mention of vaginal atrophy, as oestrogen deficiency is also a risk factor for prolapse. The type and degree of prolapse must be accurately assessed and also the contribution of coexisting prolapse, such as uterine prolapse. Any stress incontinence should be demonstrated. Advice should be given to reduce her risk of worsening prolapse, including weight reduction, stopping smoking, avoiding constipation and avoiding repetitive heavy lifting. Adequate oestrogen replacement (such as local oestrogen preparations) should be given. If the patient is asymptomatic, no further action is required. In others, discomfort or stress incontinence may lead to consideration of pelvic floor exercises, a ring or shelf pessary or operative repair. Pessaries are usually reserved for those patients who are medically unfit, as there are long-term problems with usage, such as vaginal ulceration and loss of effectiveness owing to worsening of the prolapse. Prior to operative repair, consideration should be given to detailed urodynamic investigation if this woman has urinary symptoms, particularly if she has had previous surgery or has a mixed urinary incontinence picture. If the dominant feature is that of genuine stress incontinence, then it may be appropriate to concentrate on that aspect (that is, consider suprapubic bladder neck surgery), rather than complete anatomical correction of the cystourethrocoele. An anterior colporrhaphy would be appropriate if she has discomfort and no significant urinary symptoms. Care must be taken, if she has had previous vaginal surgery or a posterior colporrhaphy is also being considered, that the vagina is not narrowed in sexually active women.

Comments
This is a GP referral of a lady who might be symptom-free, so all options should be mentioned, such as no treatment and advice, physiotherapy, ring or shelf pessary and surgery.

When discussing surgical options, mention sexual function.

Careful assessment of this woman determines management and indicates the likely treatment outcome, so demonstrate your knowledge of the symptoms and risk factors associated with prolapse, such as urinary and bowel symptoms and respiratory disease.

Suggested reading
Jeffcoate T W A, Roberts H 1952 Stress incontinence. British Journal of Obstetrics and Gynaecology 59: 685–720
Shaw R W, Soutter W P, Stanton S L (eds) 1996 Gynaecology, 2nd edn. Churchill Livingstone, Edinburgh

2. **A 40-year-old woman is found to have stage 1b carcinoma of the cervix. Describe how this staging would have been reached and critically discuss the options for management.**

Clinical staging of this stage 1b carcinoma of the cervix is performed as a formal procedure under general anaesthesia by two experienced gynaecologists. Satisfactory exposure of the upper vagina and cervix using a Simm's speculum and an appropriate vaginal wall retractor is necessary to measure the dimensions of the lesion and take an adequate biopsy. The cervical canal would be explored and curettage of both the endometrium and the endocervix is performed. Bimanual examination and palpation of the parametrium is performed to assess possible spread. Rectal examination and cystoscopy are performed to assess possible bladder or rectal involvement. Information from chest X-ray and intravenous urography is also considered. Stage 1b carcinoma of the cervix is a carcinoma confined to the uterus and as such encompasses a large range of tumour volumes. Computerised tomography or magnetic resonance imaging may consolidate the clinical picture and give information regarding lymph node involvement, but does not alter the official staging. In a young woman, provided she is medically fit and this is a small tumour with no suspicion of lymph node involvement, a radical hysterectomy with lymph node dissection is the definitive treatment. If the lymph nodes are involved, postoperative radiotherapy is offered. However, if the woman has other intercurrent illness, a larger tumour volume (over 4 cm in diameter), or is suspected of having lymph node metastasis, radiotherapy is performed as a primary treatment. A radical hysterectomy has the advantage of allowing the woman to conserve her ovaries and to maintain sexual function. In a young woman, there is also a theoretical long-term risk of a radiation-induced tumour. Radical hysterectomy is, however, a major operation with high attendant morbidity, intraoperative blood loss, risk of thromboembolism and risk of ureter, bladder and bowel injury. Voiding dysfunction secondary to bladder denervation is common. Radiotherapy causes short-term side-effects of gastrointestinal upset and radiation cystitis. More significant are the long-term side-effects of vaginal stenosis, bowel and urinary strictures and fistulae and lymphoedema. Careful preoperative counselling is an essential part of the decision-making process.

Comments
Answering gynae-oncology questions often pivots on remembering the correct staging of gynaecological malignancy. So, learn the staging and relearn it. Make sure you have the most up to date FIGO staging. Unless you have revised it thoroughly, this is the sort of information that might desert you in an examination panic. Make sure you read it within the 48 hours before the examination.

Write the actual definition of the relevant stage down at the beginning of your plan.

Suggested reading
Burghardt (ed) 1993 Surgical gynaecological oncology. Thieme Medical Publications, Stuttgart
Coppleson M 1992 Gynaecological oncology, 2nd edn. Churchill Livingstone, Edinburgh

3. Critically evaluate the role of a routine 6 week postoperative hospital visit following major gynaecological surgery.

The 6 week visit has been the cornerstone of postoperative management for many years. It is a simple and effective way to monitor patient satisfaction, to ensure that all investigations are complete and to monitor the success rate of the procedure. The visit is particularly important for audit purposes in newer and unusual procedures and those operations with success rates that are particularly operator dependent. In addition, specialist follow-up may be needed for these procedures, as the primary care team may be unaware of the potential complications. All malignancies must be followed up in the outpatients because of the need for continuing counselling, review of any outstanding results and to organise adjuvant treatment. A follow-up appointment is often required after day case surgery, as the after-effects of anaesthesia sometimes lead to poor recall of immediate postoperative counselling. A follow-up visit may also be useful to ensure tolerance and to adjust treatment started.

There are significant disadvantages, however. Routine follow-up, rather than targeted follow-up, is expensive both to the hospital and the patient. The distance travelled and expenses incurred must be justified by clear benefit, particularly in rural areas. In well-established procedures, follow-up is not required, or could be undertaken by the primary care team. The majority of hysterectomies for menorrhagia are in this category. If histology results are not available before discharge, the results could be communicated to the general practitioner. Only those with abnormal results would then require follow-up. The 6-week period is often inappropriate. Those with menstrual problems require a longer interval, whilst those awaiting histology results or to discuss operative findings should be seen sooner.

In most modern units, the routine 6 week visit is inappropriate and targeting of follow-up utilises resources more effectively. Schemes using nurse-led or primary care follow-up should be considered. Patient satisfaction and audit may be performed by questionnaire or telephone enquiry. In places where general practitioner participation is uncertain and administrative processing of results unreliable, there is still a strong case for provision of the 'safety net' 6 week appointment.

Comments
This type of question is not helped by extensive examination preparation. It only needs a common-sense approach to score highly.
The answer should be structured into the current function of the preoperative visit, criticism relating to the routine nature of the visit and the 6-week timing.

Suggested reading
Tindall V R 1990 Jeffcoate's principles of gynaecology, 5th edn.
Butterworths, London

4. A 28-year-old woman presents with her husband of 1 year's standing, having been unable to consummate their marriage. How would you manage this problem?

Ideal management of this difficult and sensitive problem requires careful exploration of the issues involved with each partner individually and then together. This should be conducted in an atmosphere of privacy, free from interruptions and with adequate time allotted. Input from experienced counsellors in this field must be sought as required. If there is marital disharmony, for example, counselling is a priority.

A full history, examination and appropriate investigations should be performed on each partner. In the male partner, previous sexual relationships, sexual orientation, loss of libido and erectile dysfunction are all important areas to be covered. There is an association of general health and sexual function. Diabetes, for example, is related specifically to impotence. Examination may reveal a specific physical problem such as a congenital penile abnormality.

In the female partner, the cause may also be psychological or physical. Exploration of previous sexual relationships, sexual orientation and history of sexual abuse is important. Loss of libido is more likely to have a psychological origin in females. Examination may reveal vaginismus or a physical barrier to intercourse. A mechanical barrier may be secondary to female genital mutilation in certain ethnic groups, or secondary to a congenital abnormality such as vaginal atresia and stenosis, or a thickened hymen.

Having established the diagnosis from the history and examination, supported by relevant investigations, treatment will then depend on the aetiology. In erectile dysfunction, it is important to effect a prompt urology referral. For psychological aetiologies in both male and female partners, involvement of a sex therapist and expert psychosexual counsellor is essential. Decreased libido may be treated with a formal programme such as the 'sensate focus' approach. Vaginismus may be treated with a programme using vaginal dilators, lubrication and culminating in intercourse in the female dominant position.

It may be necessary to examine the female partner under general anaesthesia. If there is a physical barrier, such as female genital mutilation or toughened hymen, it may be possible to correct the problem surgically. In cases of the rarer congenital abnormalities, it will be useful to seek the advice of an expert in the field.

Comments
Convey the impression that you appreciate that this is a sensitive issue and careful exploration of the history of the woman and her partner individually and together is appropriate.

The importance of the involvement of specialist help must be covered.

The causes can be classified into physical, psychological and sexual orientation.

Suggested reading
De Witt D E 1991 Dyspareunia: tracing the cause. Postgraduate
Medicine 89: 67–73
Reader F 1991 Disorders of female sexuality. In: Studd J (ed) Progress
in obstetrics and gynaecology. Churchill Livingstone, Edinburgh,
vol 9, pp 303–317
Van Lankveld J J 1995 Difficulties in the differential diagnosis of
vaginismus, dyspareunia and mixed sexual pain disorders. Journal of
Psychosomatic Obstetrics and Gynaecology 16: 201–209

5. **During routine investigations for infertility, a hysterosalpingogram
shows a hypoplastic uterus and absent right tube. Explore the
management options.**

The management options depend on an accurate assessment of the
degree of uterine abnormality in the context of the particular patient's
circumstances. Despite this obvious abnormality, assessment would
encompass a full history, examination and investigation of both patient
and partner. The degree of hypoplasia may vary in severity from a
small rudimentary single uterus to one which is approximately two-
thirds of normal size. The woman may have a history of secondary
infertility, rather than primary, proving conception is possible. A history
of a previous full-term normal delivery would indicate that the uterine
abnormality is of even less importance. Significant uterine
abnormalities are associated with recurrent miscarriage and premature
labour. Hypoplasia can be congenital or acquired secondary to a
reduction of oestrogen or a combination of the two. In this case, where
there is an absence of a fallopian tube, this would indicate a congenital
cause. There is an association with sex chromosome abnormalities,
therefore performing a karyotype of the patient would be essential.
A hormonal profile to exclude endocrine abnormality is indicated.
A laparoscopy would be required to confirm the presence of tubal
patency and identify the ovaries. The urinary system should be
investigated with an intravenous pyelogram, as the risk of a coexistent
urinary tract abnormality is in the order of 10%. Where an endocrine
abnormality is implicated, oestrogen therapy may increase the size of
the uterus, but this would be reversed on treatment cessation. It may
be considered prior to active fertility treatment. Careful counselling of
the couple is essential. In the case of a minor degree of hypoplasia, in
the absence of any other fertility problem and particularly with a history
of secondary infertility, fertility treatment may be an option. In the
absence of normal ovaries, donor oocyte in vitro fertilisation could be
considered. In less favourable circumstances, successful conception
would be unlikely, therefore adoption of a child should be explored.
Another theoretical option is surrogacy. Though in practice this is
fraught with difficulty, it may be the only option for the couple to have
their genetic child.

Comments
This is a rare congenital abnormality, but it is still essentially a subfertility
question. It is easiest to approach it from this angle.
Remember to discuss both the woman and her partner.

Note the omissions from the question: whether this is primary or secondary subfertility, the results of other investigations and details regarding the partner. Nor does the question include information regarding the severity of the hypoplasia.

Suggested reading
Johnson N, Lilford R J 1990 The surgical management of gynaecological congenital malformations. In: Studd J (ed) Progress in obstetrics and gynaecology. Churchill Livingstone, Edinburgh, vol 8, pp 351–369
Tindall V R 1990 Jeffcoate's principles of gynaecology, 5th edn. Butterworths, London

PAPER 10

1. Minimal-access surgery should replace open surgery in gynaecological practice. Critically evaluate this statement.

The revolution in fibreoptic technology over recent years has allowed rapid progress in the field of minimal-access surgery (MAS). The benefits of MAS include improved cost-effectiveness, decreased morbidity, shorter hospital stay, earlier return to work and possible better cosmetic result compared with conventional surgery.

However, MAS has limitations and cannot be regarded as interchangeable with open surgery. There are occasions in which the use of the laparoscopic approach can be considered as hazardous and the use of open surgery essential. There is the risk of visceral damage in women who have undergone multiple surgery, although open instrumentation reduces this risk. In cases of haemorrhage, rapid stabilisation of the patient and control of blood loss is the priority and is most effectively accomplished by an open procedure. Some diagnostic information is lacking in minimal-access surgery, as the tactile information is absent and gaining undisrupted histological specimens is difficult. Full surgical staging is therefore not possible laparoscopically, making the use of MAS limited in gynae-oncology. Menstrual reduction can be achieved by techniques such as transcervical resection and laser ablation of the endometrium, but patient satisfaction is lower than with hysterectomy, as the incidence of amenorrhoea is low. Hysterectomy is the preferred option in women with additional dysmenorrhoea (possible adenomyosis) or leiomyomata. Laparoscopic hysterectomy appears to have no advantage over vaginal hysterectomy and is technically difficult, requires expensive technology and is time-consuming. Laparoscopic ablation of endometriosis has been a major advance in the treatment, but often open surgery is still required.

A laparoscopic surgeon must first be experienced in open surgery as, in case of complications, the laparoscopic surgeon may need to convert to an open procedure. The wide adoption of MAS would lead to fewer cases available for open surgery training.

MAS will not replace open surgical procedures in all aspects of surgery. In only a few instances, MAS can replace open surgery, though it remains a useful option in many more cases. Careful audit and research is essential to continually re-evaluate the place of minimal-access surgery in gynaecology.

Comments

The term 'critically evaluate' means examine the evidence for and against this statement. Do not just give your view justified by appropriate evidence. That would only constitute part of the answer required.

The examiner may or may not be in favour of minimal-access surgery, but his opinion is irrelevant as he will be using a structured marking system.

Suggested reading

Shaw R W 1995 Minimal access surgery in gynaecology. Current Obstetrics and Gynaecology 5: 125

Tindall V R 1990 Jeffcoate's principles of gynaecology, 5th edn.
Butterworths, London

2. **A 20-year-old mentally retarded woman attends the clinic requesting contraceptive advice. Compare management strategies.**

Contraception is an important, but often neglected, issue in this group of women. Many mentally retarded women manage independently, but pregnancy produces an extra burden on both the woman involved and the carers. A mentally retarded woman may not be able to care for her child independently and her parents, who may be elderly, may not be able to cope with caring for a child in addition. It is essential to take a full history and perform a full examination. The reasons that prompted the visit should be explored and the details regarding social circumstances are very important. This woman apparently presented of her own volition, which indicates a degree of awareness and allows a better assessment to be made. If there is a regular sexual partner, contraception is ideally discussed with the couple together. The woman may wish sterilisation. Obtaining informed consent is difficult in this situation, so medicolegal advice should be sought and carers and next of kin involved in the counselling process. If sterilisation is performed, all parties must be aware of the slight failure risk of 1–3 per 1000, particularly in view of the increased chance of an ectopic pregnancy with failed sterilisation. Barrier contraception can be considered only in a stable relationship and as the oral contraceptive pill is intolerant of erratic administration, it must be administered by a carer. An injectable progestogen such as medroxyprogesterone acetate is an excellent choice and only requires administration every 3 months. A subcutaneous progesterone implant is effective for 5 years. Insertion and removal under local anaesthetic may be difficult if the woman is uncooperative. In a parous women, an intrauterine contraceptive device (IUCD) can be considered, or the progesterone-releasing coil (improved contraceptive effect and menstrual reduction). Progesterone injections and implants often cause irregular bleeding in the short term and the IUCD tends to cause menorrhagia. This may prove unacceptable for the woman and her carer. In women who also have menorrhagia, suitable methods include carer administered combined oral contraceptive pill or the progesterone-releasing coil. In those women with menorrhagia in whom sterilisation is planned, a hysterectomy may be considered.

Comments
Consideration of all categories of contraception must be discussed, with particular reference to the method's suitability or unsuitability in each case.
A central management problem is the difficulty in obtaining 'informed consent'. This must be discussed.
Remember to discuss the male partner!

Suggested reading
Coverdale J H 1993 Respecting the autonomy of chronic mentally ill women in decisions about contraception. Hospital Community Psychiatry 44: 671–674

Haefner H K, Elkins T E 1991 Contraceptive management for female adolescents with mental retardation and handicapping disabilities. Current Opinion in Obstetrics and Gynaecology 3: 820–824

3. **A 44-year-old woman presents with vulval soreness. Vulval colposcopy and directed biopsy confirm vulval intraepithelial neoplasia 1 (VIN I). Discuss the options for her care.**

VIN I is equivalent to mild atypia/dysplasia, which is limited to the lower third of the epithelium. The exact aetiology is unknown, but may be due to viral infection with HPV. In such a woman who presents with confirmed VIN I, the first option is to perform a full history, examination and colposcopic assessment of the genital tract and if there are no other findings, to pursue conservative management. During the examination, a coincidental cause for the vulval soreness, such as infection or atrophy (in premature menopause), should be excluded. Infection and oestrogen deficiency are thought to be implicated in the aetiology of VIN, therefore swabs for culture and sensitivity and serum luteinising hormone and follicle stimulating hormone should be taken as appropriate, in addition to a cervical smear. Immunosuppression can also be implicated in VIN and therefore must be considered. Colposcopic assessment must include careful inspection of the whole vulva, vagina, anus and cervix. VIN is often multifocal and may be part of a wider field change throughout the genital tract, so it is essential to rule out lesions in all these areas. Advice should be given regarding the risk factors implicated in VIN, including smoking. Infection must be treated and oestrogen deficiency corrected. The woman should be seen in 6 months to repeat colposcopic assessment, as there is a chance that the lesion will regress spontaneously. Colposcopy must include the cervix, as around 25% have cervical intraepithelial neoplasia. In this case, no further action should be taken, other than repeating the assessment in 12 months and then, if no recurrence is noted, the patient can be discharged back to her general practitioner. If the lesion persists, but has not progressed, close observation by regular colposcopic examination is essential on a 6-monthly basis.

If the lesion progresses to VIN II/III, definitive treatment must be considered. In an isolated small lesion, excision or laser treatment could be of value. In more extensive lesions, a simple vulvectomy may be required, although the effect on sexual function of a relatively young woman can be significant. New treatment modalities such as retinoid or interferon therapy have not been adequately evaluated.

Comments

The central concept to answering this question is that VIN is a multifocal lesion and can be part of a field change throughout the genital tract. Observation and follow-up are the mainstay of her management only once other lesions have been excluded, e.g. cervical intraepithelial neoplasia.

Remember to mention the management of the woman's complaint. Other pathology may be responsible for her symptoms.

Suggested reading
Shepherd J J, Monaghan J M 1990 Clinical gynaecological oncology, 2nd edn. Blackwell Science, Oxford

4. **A 24-year-old woman has a 2-year history of unexplained infertility. Compare and contrast the management options.**

After full counselling of the woman and her partner, the options lie between conservative management and assisted reproduction. Conservative management may be suitable for those couples who do not wish to embark on assisted reproduction, or those who are ineligible for treatment. In unexplained infertility, there is still a chance of spontaneous conception, although low. Conservative management could include monitoring of ovulation and semen analysis at agreed intervals. Further discussion regarding assisted reproduction should take place at a later date, as success rates decline significantly in females after the age of 30. The options for assisted reproduction include intrauterine insemination (IUI), in vitro fertilisation (IVF) and gamete intrafallopian transfer (GIFT). Availability is limited, particularly in the NHS. IUI is the least costly of these options. It also has the advantage of being less invasive, less technologically demanding and a less demanding time commitment for the couple. It can be performed without ovulation induction, though the success rate is thought to be lower. If ovulation induction is used, there is a risk of multiple pregnancy, although this is reduced by careful ultrasound monitoring. The success rate is lower than the other techniques. The conception rate for this technique in unexplained infertility approaches 30% for three treatment cycles. IVF has a superior success rate with a cumulative conception rate approaching 45% in some centres for three treatment cycles. The technique is costly, invasive and involves supraovulation with its attendant risks. Multiple pregnancy is common, dependent on the number of embryos transferred. GIFT is also a costly technique and involves supraovulation, but has a good success rate. It is estimated that whereas about one-fifth of women will have a child per cycle of IVF treatment, one-third will have a child per cycle of GIFT. However, it adds laparoscopy to the techniques required and therefore also a general anaesthetic, so this technique has waned in popularity.

At the age of 24, there is time to adopt a stepwise approach to the management of this couple, commencing with IUI or GIFT, followed by IVF should this initial approach be unsuccessful.

Comments
The question stipulates that the woman has unexplained infertility, so it wishes to concentrate on other management issues. Whether this is primary or secondary infertility is not mentioned.

The term 'management options' is used, not 'treatment options'. This means that 'no treatment' should be included in the discussion as an option. A broad comparison between treatment methods is all that is needed in such a specialised question.

Suggested reading
Abdalla H, Baber R, Studd J 1990 Active management of infertility.
In: Studd J (ed) Progress in obstetrics and gynaecology.
Churchill Livingstone, Edinburgh, vol 8, pp 273–287

5. **What a remarkable impact gonadotrophin releasing hormone analogues (GnRH-a) have made in gynaecology. Review their usage.**

Gonadotrophin releasing hormone (GnRH), sometimes known as LHRH, is a decapeptide hormone secreted in intermittent pulses from the hypothalamus. The synthetic GnRH analogues cannot be administered orally, only by injection or nasal spray. Synthetic, long-acting analogues of GnRH have been synthesised which, when given, will lead to pituitary desensitisation, resulting in ovarian steroidogenesis suppression. This phenomenon is the basis for treating many conditions which are gonadotrophin and/or ovarian hormone dependent. Short-term side-effects include hot flushes and skin and hair changes. The usage of GnRH analogues is time limited by the consequences of oestrogen deficiency, as long-term usage can cause osteoporosis. This problem has been partially addressed by the additional use of add-back hormone replacement therapy. The longest established gynaecological use of GnRH analogues is in the field of assisted reproduction. Down-regulation of ovarian activity is now an essential component of many assisted reproduction regimes. Their use in the treatment of endometriosis is now well established, as they produce effective medical treatment whilst being better tolerated than danazol. However, as with all medical regimes, symptoms of endometriosis often return within the year. There was much excitement regarding their potential role in reduction of the size of leiomyomata. However, following cessation of usage, the leiomyomata increase in size, making GnRH analogues ineffective treatment in their own right. However, there is evidence that their usage preoperatively can allow an easier hysterectomy and even convert an abdominal operation to the vaginal approach. When used prior to myomectomy, they cause both shrinking and reduction of vascularity, facilitating subsequent surgery. For the same reason, GnRH analogues cannot be used for long-term treatment of menorrhagia. However, they are useful to induce amenorrhoea, to allow an iron deficiency anaemia to be corrected and to thin the endometrium prior to endometrial laser ablation or resection. Other uses include the treatment of precocious puberty and the treatment of premenstrual syndrome. It has been suggested that these analogues would be effective in the treatment of oestrogen-dependent tumours such as endometrial and breast carcinoma, but further research is awaited.

Comments
'Review' is a broad type of question and unlikely to be used for a short essay title unless it is a narrow topic or the term is qualified (e.g. review critically). Try to give examples from the breadth of gynaecology, rather than focusing on one field.

Don't get carried away with a topical discussion on the merits of add-back therapy. The question is interested only in GnRH-a. A discussion of the usage of add-back HRT is only justified as part of the discussion of the side-effect profile.

As the question uses an abbreviation, you are justified in using the abbreviation from the outset in the examination. Remember to use exactly the same abbreviation, however.

Suggested reading

Flanagan C A 1997 Advances in understanding gonadotrophin releasing hormone receptor structure and ligand interactions. Reviews of Reproduction 2: 113–120

Studd J, Leather A 1996 The need for add-back with gonadotrophin releasing hormone agonist therapy. British Journal of Obstetrics and Gynaecology 103(suppl 14): 1–4

THE ORAL ASSESSMENT EXAMINATION

The Part 2 MRCOG oral assessment examination

In November 1998, the Royal College of Obstetricians and Gynaecologists introduced a new-style oral assessment examination, which replaced the clinical and oral components of the Membership examination. There is a progress mark in the written examination which candidates must achieve in order to proceed to the oral assessment examination (this mark is under continuous review). However, to pass the examination, candidates must pass the oral component and achieve an overall pass mark when the written and oral component marks are combined.

WHY CHANGE?

1. In the old-style clinical and oral examinations, because of variations in patients, the number of topics covered and examiner variability, every candidate effectively sat a different examination. This produced an examination that was low in *reliability and reproducibility.*
2. *Patients* varied in the complexity or rarity of their disease, their intelligence and their fluency in English. An inarticulate woman speaking in regional dialect with a strong accent and unfamiliar words is a challenge to native English speakers and downright unfair to overseas candidates accustomed to hearing BBC English or English as spoken in, say, India.
   It became increasingly difficult to recruit women as patients for the clinical examination, particularly in gynaecology. Fewer women were willing to be examined (especially vaginally) by doctors who were unfamiliar to them and for a purpose which did not directly benefit them, i.e. in planning their treatment. Patients, despite instruction, varied in their willingness to divulge information; some took the attitude that it was the candidate's job to discover the diagnosis with no help from them, whilst others reeled off the diagnosis, tests, results and the management plan as soon as the candidate walked into the room. How they behaved could have depended on whether they liked the candidate or not.
3. *Examiners* also varied. Some examiners asked every candidate the same question and others asked every candidate a different question. Some were 'Hawks' and others 'Doves'. Some had idiosyncrasies. Whilst the presence of a second examiner did go some way to reducing these variables, they were not eliminated.
4. The *number of topics* covered varied from as few as four (two in the clinical and two in the oral) to as many as eight, and furthermore they were chosen by the examiner.

5. In order that the examination be *fair*, every candidate would need to have seen and examined the same pair of patients with the same pair of examiners using the same criteria for marking. Alternatively, a larger number of patients per candidate (about 12) would have ironed out some of the problems by covering a greater number of topics and therefore ensuring a reasonable spread of difficult and easy patients. With about 400 candidates, these measures were impossible to achieve.

THE ORAL ASSESSMENT EXAMINATION

The oral assessment examination overcomes many of these drawbacks. Because there are the same 10 questions with the same standardised answer and marking scheme, reliability and reproducibility are improved. However, the examination is expensive to set up and time-consuming. Both candidates and examiners may be sceptical about the examination at first because they are not familiar with it. All MRCOG examiners have experience of OSCE-type examinations at undergraduate and/or DRCOG levels. Furthermore, the examiners are trained in the principles of the new examination and, on the eve of the examination, study in detail those questions with which they will be involved over the following 3 days. Candidates should endeavour to learn as much as they can about the examination before appearing. There will be courses in the UK and perhaps abroad and the candidate is strongly advised to attend. The RCOG will send out guidelines to those candidates who gain the progress mark in the written part of the examination. These questions should be practised with the candidate's tutor. Remember, this is an oral examination and candidates cannot practise by reading the questions and writing out the answers. They must interact with an 'examiner' and, where appropriate, a role player, then get feedback on their performance.

The format of the examination

The oral examination takes the form of an objective, structured, clinical examination. The examination hall will be laid out with a series of tables, each of which represents a station. The tables are usually set out in a circle or a rectangle (the circuit), depending on the shape of the room. There will be the same number of candidates as there are stations and one candidate will be seated at each table so that all the stations are occupied. At each station there is a task to be performed. After the set time interval, a bell will sound and the candidates will all move clockwise to the next station. If there are 12 stations, then after 12 time intervals all candidates will have completed the circuit and had the opportunity to answer all the questions.

In the MRCOG oral examination, there are 12 stations, but only 10 are 'active' and have an examiner present. It is at these stations that marks are awarded. Two 'preparatory' stations are included where candidates are expected to study or read some material on which they will be examined at the next station. In the example given in Figure 1, the two candidates starting at stations 2 and 8 will be taken into the hall 15 minutes before the examination proper starts, in order to study the material at stations 1 and 7 respectively. They will of course finish 15 minutes earlier than the other candidates.

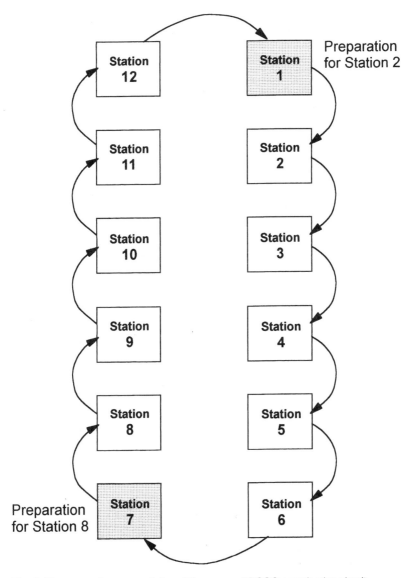

Fig. 1 Diagrammatic representation of the new oral RCOG examination circuit. *Note*: the two preparatory stations may not be evenly distributed in the circuit.

The duration of each station is 15 minutes. This is much longer than in undergraduate and DRCOG examinations, which are typically 5 and 6 minutes. This allows the candidate to perform more complicated tasks and the examiner to explore the candidate's knowledge, skill and clinical experience in greater depth. In this way, the examiner can judge whether or not the candidate is of an appropriate standard to be awarded the MRCOG.

At the end of each 15-minute period, a bell will sound and candidates will move in a clockwise direction to the next station. The examiners remain at one station for the whole session and therefore every candidate will meet the same 10 examiners. The examination will last $12 \times 15 = 180$ minutes, i.e. 3 hours. There will be a 10-minute break about halfway through the examination, when candidates and examiners will be allowed to visit the toilet. The break time will be predetermined for each circuit and candidates who leave the room at any other time will reduce the time spent at the station and are unlikely to complete the task required and will therefore lose marks. It will be prudent to empty the bladder before the examination starts. Once the examination is underway, it cannot be stopped for reasons other than an emergency such as a fire or a candidate inducing a heart attack in one of the examiners! The comfort break will of course extend the examination time by 10 minutes, i.e. 3 hours and 10 minutes in total.

The examination will be held over 3 days and there will be two sessions per day, morning and afternoon. For the first examination, November 1998, there were six circuits in each session, split between two venues, one of which was the RCOG building. Thus, there were 36 oral examination sessions in all. As the number of candidates varies, the number of circuits can be increased or decreased accordingly, but the number of stations in each circuit will, for the foreseeable future, remain constant.

Candidates will be advised in writing, in the form of an entrance card, of the day, session and venue of their examination. Also printed on the card will be the circuit and the starting station (see Fig. 2). Stewards will check that candidates are in the right place at the right time before each examination commences. Candidates will also be required to furnish proof of their identity in the form of an official document bearing a photograph and name and written in English. An example would be a passport, a hospital identification document or a driving licence (if a photograph is included).

On any one day, the questions in every circuit will be identical. Morning and afternoon candidates will not be allowed to meet. The afternoon set of candidates will be kept in a holding room whilst the morning set leaves. On the second and third days, the questions will be similar but not identical. In this way, candidates sitting on, say, Monday will not be able to help Tuesday candidates. In any case, encouraging a colleague to get a better mark may cause you to fail because of the way in which the pass mark is determined. How the examination is marked is discussed later in this chapter.

There will be a briefing session for candidates before the examination starts.

The questions

At every station there will be a sheet of paper, fastened to the desk so that the previous candidate cannot take it away, with the candidate's instructions. For example, 'Mrs X is attending your clinic today. Read the referral letter and then ask Mrs X any questions you think appropriate in

---

ROYAL COLLEGE OF OBSTETRICIANS AND GYNAECOLOGISTS
27 Sussex Place , Regent's Park, London NW1 4RG
Telephone +44 (0) 171 etc.

MEMBERSHIP EXAMINATION

Dr Pamela Buck   Candidate No: 12345

REGISTRATION
The registration desk will be open from (time) am to (time) am. Please ensure you have registered by (time) am. Candidates that are late will not be admitted.

Address for registration
RCOG
27 Sussex Place
Regent's Park
London
NW1 4RG

ORAL EXAMINATION

Date: Monday 16 November 1998

Session: AM   Circuit: B   Starting Station No: 10

This card must be brought to the examination together with evidence of identification which must show your name and photograph (e.g. passport, hospital identification card, etc.)

Dr P Buck
St Mary's Hospital
Whitworth Park
MANCHESTER
M13 0JH

                                              LONDON
                                              RCOG

Fig. 2 Sample entry card.

order to reach a diagnosis'. The next station might read, 'Discuss with the examiner what investigations you would perform on Mrs X and how you might manage her gynaecological problem'. What exactly is being tested at the station will also be indicated, e.g. 'At this station you will be awarded marks for taking a history'.

1. Critical reading

A document will be placed at a preparatory station and the candidate is expected to read and study it, then answer questions on it at the next 'active' station. The document could be a scientific paper, an information leaflet designed either for patients, midwives or doctors, or promotional literature for a new drug. A video could also be appraised in the same way.

The sort of questions that might be asked could include:

- Is the document written appropriately for the target reader?
- Is the information incomplete or too detailed or confusing?
- Is the content accurate or misleading?
- Is the study design appropriate?
- Is there a control group and is it appropriate?
- Are there any statistical errors which lead to the wrong conclusion being drawn?
- Was the project worthwhile? Does it have practical applications for clinical practice? Does it make significant advances in medical science?

Clearly, which questions are asked will depend on the document. Candidates will be expected to appraise the document with a critical mind and not just take its contents at face value. The instructions will be given at that station and will make it clear what they are expected to do. On reaching the real station, the examiner will repeat the instructions then ask specific questions relating to the document. The examiner will already have studied it so he/she understands the questions and their significance.

2. Consultation skills

The 'patient' at this type of station is a professional actor. Like most actors, they work from a script provided by the question setter. They will have rehearsed their role in advance so that their responses and body language are appropriate.

The actor may portray a patient, a relative or a fellow professional: midwife, nurse or doctor.

Candidates will be asked to do any one of a number of tasks depending on the clinical scenario.

Taking a history. The questions asked of the patient must be relevant to her complaint, e.g. whether or not she has an outside toilet may be appropriate for a complaint of urgency of micturition but not for pelvic pain. If a general anaesthetic may be involved in your management, enquiry about her cardiorespiratory fitness should be included. If antibiotic therapy is an option, hypersensitivity reactions should be asked about. Time should not be wasted asking irrelevant questions. There are only 15 minutes and the history taking will be only one component. Time must be allowed to complete the rest of the question: perhaps a discussion about the management which will involve examination of the patient, investigations and possibly several treatment options.

Communicating information. The candidate may be asked to read some information about a patient or her complaint and then discuss it with her. Alternatively, the patient may have read about a new technique in the press. The candidate will be asked to discuss the pros and cons of the technique with her: it may or may not be appropriate.

Counselling. The patient may present enquiring about, say, contraception. Candidates will need to find out her particular needs and circumstances and if there are any contraindications to certain methods. There should follow a discussion on the various methods to help her make a decision. Note that counselling means assisting her to make a choice or decision, by discussing the options and relating them to her circumstances. It does not mean telling her what to do.

Breaking bad news. The candidate will be given some information about a patient and will be expected to tell her sensitively and sympathetically. It may be that she has been found to have an advanced carcinoma of the cervix at examination under anaesthesia or that her fetus has been found to have a serious abnormality on ultrasound.

Whenever there is a patient at a station, marks will be given for communication skills and not just for knowledge of her condition. Proper and professional introduction is required: 'Good morning Mrs Smith, I am Dr Buck, the consultant', and not 'Hi! I'm Pam'. Worse still is no introduction at all. If the patient is a lay person, everyday language should be used and not medical terms, e.g. passing urine instead of micturition. The candidate should listen to what she has to say and not interrupt. Candidates' questions can be asked when she has finished and the patient invited to ask questions at each stage of the consultation. A useful technique is to ask her to repeat in her own words what she has been told. This will ensure that she has understood. The candidate should not stare at the documents or notes, but look at her, maintain eye contact and make sure facial expressions and body language are appropriate, e.g. if she is wearing a silly hat, it would be inappropriate to laugh, grin or giggle if she were being told bad news.

3. Data interpretation
At such stations, clinical or laboratory data may be given to interpret, or an X-ray, scan photograph, cytology or histology slide given to identify and then apply to a given clinical situation. If the candidate gets the diagnosis wrong, for example saying that the cytology slide shows fungal hyphae when it actually shows severe dyskaryosis, marks will be lost for that component of the question, but the examiner will give the correct diagnosis in order that the rest of the question is sensible. Thus a discussion about antifungal therapy would be avoided and mention of colposcopy, biopsy, etc. would gain further marks.

4. Knowledge
Knowledge is primarily tested in the MCQ examination and candidates with insufficient knowledge will not proceed to the oral examination. However, some components of the oral examination require application of the candidate's knowledge. Discussion of treatment with a patient is not possible if the candidate does not know what the treatment for her disease is. There will be no purely factual stations in this examination, which is designed to test clinical skills.

5. Prioritisation
One of the skills required of a competent obstetrician and gynaecologist is the ability to decide the priority in which either patients or multiple disorders

in one patient should be dealt with, e.g. the outcome is better if pressure is applied to a bleeding laceration before transferring the casualty to hospital. In the examination, the situations will be more complicated than this, but candidates will be expected to decide what to do first and what can be left when presented with a busy labour ward and a ruptured ectopic just arrived in the accident and emergency department.

6. Operation techniques

Whilst candidates will not be expected to perform an operation on a live patient (or even a cadaver), there are now available a wide range of models used for surgical training. To be examined on the ability to perform a surgical procedure on such a model is a real possibility! Marks will be awarded for technique, on 'talking the examiner through it' as if he/she were being taught, avoidance of common complications and ability to deal with them should they arise. For example, the position of the second port in laparoscopic surgery to gain maximum mechanical flexibility whilst avoiding the inferior epigastric artery. Candidates will be expected to know and justify the choice of incision, suture materials and closure technique and may be asked to demonstrate them in a given operative situation. All candidates should know about obstetrical and gynaecological instruments and how to use them correctly and safely. Cardiopulmonary resuscitation (adult and neonatal) should not just be read up. A demonstration will be expected in the examination.

7. Physical examination

Similarly, the examination of real patients is not feasible in this context. Models of both obstetric and gynaecological patients may be used to test the ability to elicit physical signs.

Reminder! This is a clinical examination. Candidates will not pass if they have read it in a book; they will pass if they have done it properly in their everyday clinical work and reproduce their mental, manual and communication skills on the day of the examination.

Marking

The members of the oral examination subcommittee set the questions and decide on the correct answers.

There are usually two or more components to each question, one of which may carry more marks than the others. For example, if the question is designed to examine communication skills, then the majority of the marks will be awarded for this. There may, however, be some marks for giving correct information to the patient. In this way, the candidate who reassures the patient with a terrifically good bedside manner, when faced with a pathology report describing an undifferentiated carcinoma which has invaded all the way to the serosal surface, will not get the maximum marks.

No matter how many components there are, the total for any one station is 10. Part marks will be rounded down to the nearest whole number. The total for the examination is 100.

During the examination, the examiner will have in front of him/her a number of mark sheets with one sheet for each candidate. He/she will tick off the items answered correctly, indicate those omitted or wrong and make a brief note on the performance, indicating the good and bad aspects of the candidate's performance. At the end of the 15 minutes, he/she will add up the marks for that candidate and enter them on a master sheet. This sheet will have the marks of all the candidates seen at that station during that session. The mark sheet is read optically later the same day, and all the marks and totals for all candidates will be recorded and stored on computer. A printed version will be prepared for the examiners' meeting, where the pass/fail decisions are made.

Index